RISING
ABOVE

RISING ABOVE

OUR TRANSFORMATIONAL JOURNEY
TO WHOLENESS AFTER BREAST CANCER

GILLIAN LICHOTA

AND OTHER CONTRIBUTING AUTHORS

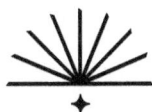

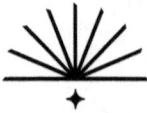

Published and distributed by Soul Speak Press.
Alexandria, USA

Library of Congress Control Number: 2025913767
Lichota, Gillian
Rising Above: Our Transformational Journey to Wholeness After Breast Cancer

ISBN
Paperback 978-1-958472-23-1
eBook 978-1-958472-24-8

To the women who gathered here—
who cracked open, bled truth onto the page, and dared to rise—
this book is your altar.

To those who came before—
we carry your memory like a sacred drumbeat.

To those yet to come—
may these words be your lantern, your tide, your map home.

This is our invocation.
This is our rising—together.

✳

To my beloved children, Kailen Jackson and Laykelyn Rielle-Cree—
You are the sacred tide that brought me back to shore. Through you, I
remembered: I was never lost, merely becoming.
You are my breath, my compass, and the light that guided me home.

✳

And to "Her Deepness," Dr. Sylvia Earle—Thank you for being the first to
show me that the ocean could hold both science and soul.
In you, I saw not just a marine explorer, but a reflection of the fearless
woman I longed to become.
Your path illuminated mine, and your voice stirred something wild and
wondrous within me.
This offering carries salt and starlight in your honor.

CONTENTS

FOREWORD

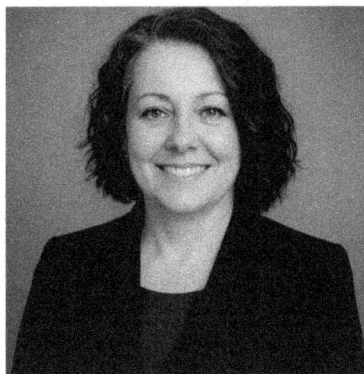

As a breast cancer survivor myself, I understand the profound impact of sharing our stories. The journey through diagnosis, treatment, and recovery is deeply personal, yet it is in these shared experiences that we find strength, hope, and community. I believe that by normalizing conversations around breast cancer and removing the stigma, we can educate and empower women at younger ages—before they ever receive a diagnosis, before they ever realize the importance of vigilance in their self-checks.

A mammogram is not recommended until the age of forty, yet breast cancer is affecting women at much younger ages. Too often, young women have not substantiated the need for self-awareness because the conversation has not yet reached them. This book seeks to change that. It is a collection of voices that speak to the realities of breast cancer, the resilience of those who endure it, and the hope that carries us forward.

The process of writing and self-exploration is healing. I am grateful to have been part of this journey, helping the women in this book share their experiences and, in doing so, providing them with a means of healing. When I was introduced to Gillian through another writer, I immediately knew we shared a mutual passion for healing through storytelling. This project is more than a book—it is a beacon of hope. I cannot wait to see *Rising Above: Our Transformational Journey to Wholeness After Breast Cancer* in every waiting room across the country, offering comfort and solidarity to those who need it most.

Storytelling has the power to remind us that we are not alone. During times of crisis, we often find ourselves in survival mode, unable to look ahead and envision the possibilities that lie beyond the struggle. But the stories within this anthology shine a light on hope, compassion, and resilience. They create opportunities for learning, for finding community, and for drawing strength from the experiences of others. In moments that feel hopeless, these stories remind us of the perseverance and fortitude that exist within us all.

This book is a lifeline for those unfamiliar with the journey, for those in need of inspiration, and for those seeking reassurance that they are not alone. To date, an anthology dedicated to the resilient women who have fought this battle has not been published—until now. This work provides a platform for healing, for connection, and for recognizing the unwavering strength of those who walk this path.

At the heart of this project is Gillian Lichota, the founder of the iRise Above Foundation, an incredible writer, and the capstone of this anthology. Her story reflects the true essence of rising through the storm—becoming a phoenix in the face of adversity. Her experience, along with the experiences of so many others, illuminates the courage it takes to navigate this journey.

Readers of this book will not only feel connected to a community but will also see the incredible support that exists throughout treatment and beyond. The journey through breast cancer is emotional and layered with complexity. These stories are not just about cancer and treatment; they are stories of compassion, hope, resilience, motherhood, the intricacies of relationships, and the unwavering dedication of our caregivers.

May this book serve as a source of strength, understanding, and hope for all who turn its pages.

—Carmen Johnson
Survivor, Advocate, and Board Member of Carolina Breast Friends

INTRODUCTION

Breast cancer is often viewed as a disease that affects older individuals—something that arises after careers are established, identities are formed, and families are nurtured. However, for the women in these pages, cancer appeared early. It struck while they were building their careers, falling in love, discovering themselves, or stepping into motherhood. It did not wait until life was settled. Instead, it shattered their expectations and disrupted their timelines. In doing so, it compelled them to awaken.

This anthology arose from that rupture—a tidal fracture that pulled us beneath the surface, only to teach us how to breathe differently.

At thirty-four, I was expecting my first child when I learned I had breast cancer. Instead of relishing this joyous occasion, I felt as though I was falling apart. The shocking realization of my own mortality while nurturing new life created a deep fracture within me, marking the beginning of my decline—or so I thought!

Years later, after the birth of my second child, cancer returned—this time metastatic and incurable. My world collapsed under the weight of grief, fear, and unresolved trauma. This ordeal compelled me to confront every hidden sorrow and cherished dream I had suppressed.

As I fell apart, writing became my sanctuary and gateway to healing—a thread of light I followed out of the darkness. It was more than catharsis; it was resurrection. I came across words that sliced through the fog of my grief like a sacred bell: "You gotta resurrect the deep pain within you and give it a place to live that's not within your body. Let it live in art. Let it live in writing. Let it live in music. Let it be devoured by building brighter connections. Your body is not a coffin for pain to be buried in. Put it somewhere else." These words by Ehime Ora shattered the illusion that I had to carry my pain alone. They offered permission—and a mandate—to alchemize suffering into expression. I understood, in that moment, that if I continued to bury the pain inside me, it would consume me. I had to transmute it, give it form, give it breath. Writing became the sacred vessel through which I turned anguish into offering, survival into voice, and breakdown into transformation.

Those words did more than illuminate my grief—they gave it direction. They reminded me that healing was not a solitary act but a sacred reclamation that required space, voice, and community. I knew I could no longer carry this burden alone. I needed a place for my pain to land—somewhere it could be witnessed, held, and transfigured. That longing for a container beyond my journal, beyond my body, became the seed of something far greater than myself.

In 2017, I founded the iRise Above Foundation. What began as a lifeline has quickly transformed into a movement. iRise Above goes beyond being just a nonprofit; it serves as a sanctuary that sparks transformation. This organization offers a refuge for young women facing breast cancer, enabling them to feel seen, supported, and in control of their healing journey. Our mission empowers these young women to overcome challenges and lead extraordinary lives—emotionally, spiritually, and physically. We envision a world where no young woman faces breast cancer alone.

As I listened to the stories of other women navigating similar devastation, I realized that this movement was never meant to carry my voice alone. What began as a personal reckoning evolved into a collective calling. I was not the only one seeking meaning in the ruins; I was one of many. Together, we were building something sacred. This anthology became the next vessel—a way to gather our stories not just to bear witness, but to offer a map—a beacon of light—for others finding their way through the dark.

At the heart of our approach is a profound conviction: Healing doesn't come from erasing pain, but from embracing and transforming it. We're committed to posttraumatic growth, the wisdom of feminine perspectives, and the power of sacred sisterhood. We believe survivorship isn't the end of the story, but the beginning of a new path toward personal growth and transformation.

At iRise Above, we focus not on repairing what is damaged but on cherishing what is sacred. We respect women in their entirety: body, mind, spirit, and soul. We create spaces where sadness and happiness can coexist, where silence is complemented by song, and where healing is cherished rather than rushed. Here, connection exists as a form of communion, woven through shared rituals, stories, and sisterhood. Empowerment means reclaiming voice, agency, and identity. We believe resilience is found not only in determination but also in grace—the gentleness that endures. What is wholeness? It's not about being pain-free but about the golden thread that weaves light through every seam. Every woman who enters this space is seen not as broken, but as a masterpiece in the process of assembly.

From these origins, the Rising Above Anthology Project was born.

This book transcends being just a collection of cancer stories; it represents a constellation of transformation. Each narrative serves as a sacred artifact, crafted through hardship and enriched with significance. The women featured here did more than survive their diagnosis; they entered the crucible and emerged renewed. Following the essence of kintsugi—the Japanese technique of mending broken pottery with gold—they embraced their flaws instead of discarding them. Each scar is a mark of honor, and every crease a shining symbol of resilience. They did not revert to their former selves; instead, they evolved into something greater: vessels of beauty, made radiant by their struggles. Their stories shine not in spite of the damage, but because of the golden rivers that now course through them. This represents not only rebirth but also renewal. This is more than survival; it is sacred reconstruction.

For each woman in this collection, cancer shattered the façade of control. It reopened old wounds and brought forth ancestral grief. Yet, it also created space for something sacred to emerge. In the rising swell of grief, they found their voice. In the undertow of sorrow, they surrendered. And in the depths, where no one could rescue them, they remembered how to swim. These women do not revert to their former selves; instead, they rise to who they were always destined to be—more radiant, more liberated, and more complete.

They are the ones who stitch souls together. They carry the torch of truth. These truth-tellers do not simply exist; they transform. Their writing was not for accolades—it was to preserve memory. They wrote to bring things back to life.

This book is their offering.

This book is for everyone—whether you are a woman newly diagnosed, a caregiver walking beside them, a loved one seeking to understand, or a soul yearning to grasp the unfathomable. Within these pages, you will encounter grief and rage, and experience grace and resilience. You will witness the unveiling—the raw, unfiltered reality of breaking down and being reborn. While it focuses on breast cancer, this book extends well beyond the diagnosis. It speaks of awakening, shedding the armor of survival to embrace radical authenticity. It is about returning to the *Self*—not as she existed before the rupture, but as she was always meant to be: whole, radiant, and undeniably alive.

To the courageous women whose voices resonate on these pages: You have not only survived; you have evolved. You haven't just expressed your pain—you have presented it as a source of healing. You are the leaders of transformation. Each story is a beacon passed to the next woman, guiding her through the shadows. You create a sacred ripple effect.

And to you, dear reader, may this book resonate with you at your current stage in life. May it act as a soothing balm, a reflective mirror, and a guiding beacon. If you're newly diagnosed, may you find solace in these supportive sisterly voices. If you're a caregiver, may these narratives shed light on what often remains unsaid. If cancer hasn't impacted your life, may your compassion continue to flourish. Remember, healing isn't about returning to what once was; it's about evolving into something entirely new.

Just as whales surface to breathe, just as women submerge and rise through the waters of baptism, and just as mountains emerge after the Earth shakes—you too are invited to return. Not to what was, but to who you truly are.

This is your sacred invitation to rise. This is your homecoming.

With reverence, fire, and unwavering love,
Gillian Lichota
Founder, iRise Above Foundation
Lead Author, Rising Above Anthology Project

GILLIAN LICHOTA

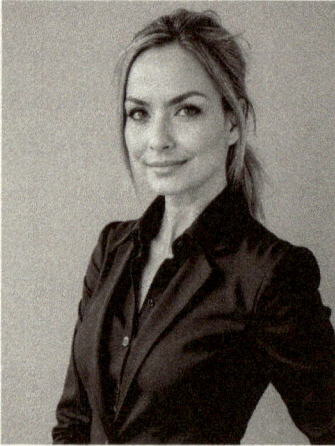

My oncologist delivered the words that every breast cancer patient dreads:

"Your cancer is back. It's metastatic—stage 4. It has spread. There is no cure."

The diagnosis struck like lightning—swift, searing, and inescapable. Time collapsed. I dropped to my knees under the weight of mortality. A storm erupted—denial, terror, sorrow, and rage—all howling through the hollow chambers of my being. I remember only one thing—echoing like a curse in the dark:

YOU-ARE-GOING-TO-DIE.

The veil between life and death thinned. I stood barefoot at its edge. And then—something ancient stirred. A voice rose—not from outside, but from my marrow:

NOT YET, GILLIAN.

My journey wasn't ending. The path split, calling me into the sacred unknown.

THE ALCHEMY OF BECOMING

Reclaiming My Voice, Body, and Light

Baptism by Fire and Water

Naked, with my head rolled back and eyes wide shut, I stood invisibly cocooned in everything I sought to control. Tears streamed down my face as a toxic mix of emotions swirled into a fierce hurricane within.

The pounding of my heartbeat drowned out the fluorescent lights. A panic attack unfolded. Water dripped from my belly onto the cold changing room floor, while humid, chlorine-laden air breezed over me from a nearby vent. I didn't recognize myself in the mirror. Eight months pregnant, my body felt like a contradiction—full of life and death. I was thin, bald, and one-breasted—physical scars of a battle etched into my flesh. Chemotherapy ended not with relief, but with profound exhaustion. Ahead lay the miracle of birth, shrouded in mystery—a threshold between life and loss, where I stood suspended between becoming a mom and fading into memory.

Burdened by guilt and shame over my newborn inheriting my illness, I whimpered, wishing to awaken from this nightmare. Then, I heard her—as if summoned from the dark recesses of my memory.

"Failure! Gillian, you ruin everything!" My mother's harsh, booming voice reverberated—loud, relentless, and all too familiar. I flinched, not just from the memory, but from the pain of wondering if she might be right.

Fearful, broken, and unsure, I asked, *How did I end up here?* And, more importantly, *How can I make this right?*

I opened my eyes to see a perfectly groomed woman watching me from across the lockers. Her long hair, flawless figure, perfectly plump breasts, and apologetic expression caught me off guard—jealousy surged through me.

I didn't realize my anger was a disguise—a shield for a truth too painful to name. I didn't resent her. I resented what she represented: completeness, control, and potential.

That day, something began to fray. The reckoning had begun.

Standing over the pool, it reflected my brokenness. I saw how control had anchored me—how chaos embodied everything I feared. I believed that exposing my fears, like shadow puppets, would make them less intimidating. However, naming them gave them life. The more I tried to control them, the more they eluded me. The shadows elongated, spreading into every aspect of my life. By attempting to contain fear, I unwittingly created a stage for it. Cancer, infertility, and betrayal took center stage.

Reflecting on my life was painful: I wasn't where I wanted to be. For years, I chased a dream of how life should be and who I was meant to become, never stopping to ask myself what *I* truly wanted. I just kept going, striving, and performing—until the illusion cracked.

Life became a dance I watched from the sidelines—close enough to ache for, yet never close enough to join.

I searched longingly for my place in the world, never realizing that the map had been inside me all along.

It became clear that I was the one holding myself back. I began to recognize the self-destructive habits that no longer served me, yet I continued to repeat them. I truly wanted to change, but fatigue made me cling to what was causing me pain.

Then, gradually, a truth emerged: *What if surrender isn't about giving up, but finding the freedom I'd been looking for all along?*

I believed time was abundant—that dreams could wait. Time felt endless—until I turned thirty-four, when cancer loomed and motherhood approached. I sensed the clock ticking in my bones. I grieved spending so little time in the present. Too many moments slipped by, lost in my pursuit of a moving target. Each day revealed the same truth: I had been playing small, settling for scraps, and starving my soul.

I avoided the sacred call to live and write my truth. A chasm grew between the life I lived and the truth I carried—wide enough to paralyze me. I clung to everything—plans, people, and outcomes—ignoring the trust buried inside me. Letting go terrified me. So, I remained cloaked in familiar darkness, wrapped in the armor of anger.

Anger was my oldest ally—sharp, loyal, and ever-ready. I wore it like a sword and a shield, convinced that the world had wronged me. But the truth? My rage wasn't about them. It was about the life I hadn't lived and the dreams fear told me to delay.

My anger didn't simmer—it splintered into sharp edges, forging armor made of impossible expectations. I hid behind perfection, polishing surfaces while burying my raw self beneath. I clung to performance like a lifeline—not addicted to substances, but to the euphoric high of achievement.

At work, I allowed no softness. At home, I feared that one crack would shatter everything. I thought control would save me—never realizing it was what confined me.

Armor is heavy. Silence corrodes. I carried invisible burdens—unspoken expectations that weighed me down. In my relationships, I gave too much and asked too little, mistaking endurance for genuine love.

My anger stemmed from the gap between who I was and who I pretended to be. Strength, I would learn, isn't about being invincible; it's about being authentic. My anger didn't boil over; it wore me down, bit by bit, until I couldn't recognize myself beneath all the striving. What remained wasn't a failure, but a woman finally tuning in beneath the noise.

My bitterness was grief in disguise—the ache of living a life that no longer fit. I had built something that appeared whole, but was stitched together from necessity, not joy. What I longed for was liberation: to crack the shell I'd outgrown and step into a more authentic self. But first, I had to surrender and risk becoming someone freer, wilder, and untamed.

To share my healing journey, I had to follow the pilgrimage that led me here—through motherhood, longing, and loss.

Motherhood is a prickly yet golden thread woven into my being—sometimes tender, sometimes barbed—always sacred. It sparked my spiritual awakening, with cancer serving as both a teacher and a torch.

My life has become a tapestry of both radiant and ragged moments, each shaping me in ways that smooth paths never could. I have been forged by fire and grace. Along the way, I've conversed with every version of myself: the frightened inner child yearning for safety and love; the furious teenager craving justice and aching to be heard; and the woman I am today—no longer running, but walking beside her shadow.

I no longer seek to silence or sever my pieces; I long to gather them and bring all of me into the light.

Becoming a mother was both a profound fear and a deep longing, shaped by my childhood scars. Determined to live differently, I pursued success as if it were a matter of survival. Each achievement became a brick in the façade I believed would protect me from my past.

I earned a full-ride scholarship to a top university, graduated with honors, built a fulfilling career, created a beautiful home, and married my best friend Boe. With every milestone, I thought I was rewriting my story. However, I overlooked a critical truth: Loving someone—especially a child—requires cultivating safety within ourselves so our wounds don't become theirs to carry.

I meticulously wove the fabric of my life with care—education, career, relationships, home—all stitched together to create an image of wholeness. Yet the one thing I longed for most—motherhood—remained out of reach.

When I finally stepped onto that path, I was met not with joy but with silence. Infertility struck like grief, drowning my hopes in sorrow too raw for words.

My body's refusal to conceive felt like betrayal—a quiet rebellion from within. Each negative test chipped away at the fragile belief that pain had a limit. It was as if the universe held up a mirror, revealing old wounds magnified through this aching void.

Shame returned like a ghost. Insecurity flared like wildfire. I spiraled into self-blame, haunted by a voice that insisted this was punishment. Outwardly, I cloaked myself in composure, layering strength over sorrow. But inside, I was unraveling—grief seeping through the seams, whispering, *"You're not enough."*

I coped by compartmentalizing pain—tucking it into boxes labeled *Later, Safe, Not Now.* I stacked them carefully around my heart, sealing them shut with achievements and the illusion of control. But infertility struck like an earthquake. The boxes buckled, lids blew off, and grief spilled out in waves. Buried memories resurfaced, and wounds I thought had healed echoed through my body.

During my first year in college, I met a charming guy who made me feel seen. However, the truth was that safety was merely an illusion. Beneath his charm, a predator lurked. When he turned on me and lashed out violently because I didn't give him something that wasn't his to have, I felt paralyzed. My body went into fear mode, and I dissociated to survive.

Though I was nineteen, I felt as if I were nine again—pulled back into a harrowing moment when my body was no longer mine, merely a battleground in an unwinnable war I couldn't stop. I hovered above myself like smoke from a burning house. My mind searched through the wreckage for some kind of anchor, magic, or a sacred word to make sense of it all.

Afterward, I collapsed inward. Shame spread like ink in water, staining everything. I didn't just feel broken—I felt contaminated. Self-blame seeped into my pores. I spun a cocoon of falsehoods to survive, convinced I was the problem—that I was too much or not enough—that I somehow invited it, deserved it, caused it. The violence left more than scars; it carved a wound into my womb. I felt defiled, hollow, and unlovable. Trauma shaped how I navigated the world. Years later, I realized its weight influenced everything—how I armored myself, how I apologized, and how I mistook surviving for healing.

Years passed. I buried the trauma under layers of achievement, pretending it hadn't left its mark. When I was finally ready to become a mother, I thought the path would clear—hadn't I demonstrated my resilience? Hadn't I paid my price in pain? But this time, my body pushed back. It remained silent, month after painful month. Fertility treatments came and went, each one flooding me with hormones and false hope—each ending in heartbreak.

After three brutal years and a second-trimester miscarriage, I finally became pregnant. It felt like a long-awaited miracle—a prayer answered. But even miracles, I would learn, can come with shadows.

What should have been a joyful celebration unraveled into a nightmare. As I carried new life inside me, another presence grew—a lump in my breast. I tried to convince myself it was nothing, but deep down I knew. The same hormones that fueled my pregnancy were feeding something sinister. The diagnosis brought my darkest fear to life: cancer growing alongside my unborn child. In creating life, I had awakened a threat that could end mine.

My body was a sanctuary, a home to two opposing forces—life and death. My womb was both a cradle and a fault line, a place where I felt joy and guilt with every ultrasound. How could I feel happy about my unborn child's heartbeat when my own mortality throbbed constantly in my chest?

I believed motherhood would be redemptive—a holy rewrite of what I had never received. But now I feared that I was passing down pain, not just love. This grief was not mine alone—it was ancestral. If I were to bring this child into the world, I would have to do what once felt impossible: become the protector I never had. I needed to nurture the child within me before I could be a mother to my unborn child.

So, the journey inward began.

Ashes of the Girl Who Disappeared

My childhood didn't unfold—it fractured. Like stained glass dropped before the light could pass through, its brilliance never fully formed. By the age of four, I began piecing together a version of myself built for survival, not play. I attuned myself to the volatile weather patterns of my parents' emotional states, forecasting their moods like a child meteorologist, hoping to outrun the storm.

They battled their demons—mental illness, addiction, despair—while I stood on the sidelines, exchanging innocence for vigilance. My mother Violet danced with shadows as her mind unraveled. My father Ricardo drowned in drink, too numb to see my fragile world eroding. Amid their chaos, I became both compass and caretaker. There was no room for me.

Neglect forced me to grow up too soon. I wore adulthood like an oversized coat, dragging its hem through the fragile landscape of my childhood while pretending it fit and, in reality, buckling beneath its weight. Anger became my shield. Boundaries vanished. Responsibility pulsed like a second heartbeat—constant, demanding, and heavy. Parentification ran deep: the need to control, the fear of failure, and a guilt that clung to me whenever I dared to prioritize myself.

During my adolescence, I longed for warmth, safety, and unconditional love from my mother—but instead, I faced Violet's explosive temper.

I became the target of her rage—her words acted as weapons, forged with precision and cruelty, each syllable piercing me like shards of glass.

I watched from the shadows of the hallway as she extended tenderness to strangers, arms wide for lovers—but never for me.

Sometimes, Violet confined me to the basement—a damp, windowless space where the walls closed in like clenched fists. I learned to be small, silent, and invisible. Every creak of the floorboards above sent my pulse racing. Through the keyhole, I watched the kitchen descend into chaos: lines of white powder carved across the counter, wild laughter erupting, bottles clinking, plastic rustling—my lullaby of dysfunction. Her face flickered between ecstasy and despair—eyes wide yet unseeing, lost in something too vast to name.

And there I was too—hovering, disembodied, and caught in the undertow of her unraveling.

I mistook her inability to care for herself as proof that I was unworthy of love.

My father Ricardo was a labyrinth of contradictions—charisma and chaos, presence and absence, warmth and wildfire. His laughter could fill a room, but behind the brightness lay a darkness that swallowed everything. His greatest devotion was to the bottle; I always came second.

Ricardo's drunken charm rendered him unpredictable—an emotional landmine I learned to tiptoe around. I never knew which version of him I'd encounter: the Joker or the Storm. His volatility forced me into the role of caretaker far too early. I was a child "parenting" her parent, cleaning up his messes—both physical and emotional—with trembling hands.

I scavenged for dignity in Ricardo's disheveled house, tidying beer bottles and cigarette ash while calculating which groceries I could afford with stolen money from my grandparents' rainy-day fund. Shame clung to me like a second skin.

Ricardo dragged me to smoke-filled parties, where rooms were thick with the pungent smell of marijuana that stung my lungs and blurred my vision. I was a child drowning in adult vices—out of place, out of breath. My legs barely reached the pedals as I slid behind the wheel—yes, the wheel—driving us home when Ricardo couldn't. I was a ghost in his world, drifting through the chaos he created. Never anchored. Never safe. Always vulnerable. Still, I stayed close, hoping one version of Ricardo might finally see me.

He drank to numb his pain; I tried to numb mine by fixing him. But what I didn't understand then was that you can't heal someone who is still pouring from an empty bottle. In the process, I began to dissolve. Quietly, I disappeared.

Even in the dimly lit basement, a spark ignited. I stumbled upon a tattered copy of *National Geographic* buried beneath a pile of old coats. The cover featured a woman floating underwater, fearless and surrounded by light. Her name—Dr. Sylvia Earle—stayed with me like a promise.

That magazine became my portal—her image—my lifeline. She dove deep while I withered in silence. I gave birth to my alter ego: *Gill Cousteau*, a nod to the legendary ocean explorer Jacques—a dream I dared to whisper. Gill wasn't afraid of the dark. She represented freedom and belonged to the sea—where nothing could hurt her, no one disappeared, and she was finally safe.

Gill Cousteau didn't just offer refuge from the dark—she carried the memory of light. She became my secret, my wildness. More than an escape—she was a prophecy—a saltwater soul holding the promise of who I'd become.

But even Gill couldn't shield me from everything. When I surfaced from our imagined depths, the reality of my home remained unchanged—chaotic, lonely, and unpredictable. To survive it, I regrettably had to become someone else.

Tethered to Violet's turmoil and Ricardo's silence, I exiled my feelings. I mastered the art of hiding, pleasing, and surviving. Approval became my currency. I didn't just fear rejection—I internalized it. I watched other mothers adore their daughters and wondered why I felt invisible. I longed to be Violet's pride and joy. Instead, I was the discarded.

That hunger for love transformed into perfectionism—and with it, an obsession with control. Chaos was my origin story. Order seemed like the only remedy.

Parentification taught me to read a room before I could read a book. My eyes scanned for danger. My breath learned to hide. I wore responsibility like a sacred charm, believing that if I held everything tightly enough, I might earn love. I mistook vigilance for virtue. When it failed me, I turned inward—building walls instead of wings. I became the one who fixed everything except herself.

The cost was a quiet ache: the belief that love must be earned through endurance, not through belonging.

But unburdening the child was just the beginning. My grief wasn't just emotional—it became cellular. My body absorbed every unmet need, silenced scream, and skipped heartbeat of love withheld. What once protected me—vigilance, control, silence—began to erode me from within. Illness became the language through which my body demanded to be heard.

Each symptom was a message—unhealed grief made flesh, whispering truths I had long buried. I could no longer dismiss the signals. My body wasn't betraying me; it was trying to liberate me. What once helped me survive had become too heavy to carry.

Gill Cousteau was born in darkness, but she was never meant to remain there. She was a thread of light, a salt-stained compass guiding me back to something sacred: The water, yes—but more than that, to the part of me that remembered how to flow, breathe, and feel. The ocean would one day gather all my broken pieces and return them whole.

I wasn't running from trauma anymore. I was swimming toward truth—reclaiming the part of me that already knew how to survive, and now was ready to rise.

When the Body Becomes the Oracle

I entered recovery the same way I lived: with clenched fists, laser focus, and a refusal to come undone. Endurance was my default; softness was an afterthought. Healing wasn't a sanctuary—it was a conquest. Pain wasn't felt; it was filed and cataloged beneath the label of *Survival.*

Control was my creed. Achievement was my altar. After childbirth, treatment, and surgery, I returned to my career as a marine biologist without pause—unshakable on the surface, polished, and productive. But rigidity had become my life raft. Beneath it, I surrendered joy, peace, and presence to the gods of performance. Applause became armor. I mistook admiration for protection.

But armor doesn't mend what it hides. Beneath the applause lived a girl shaped by chaos. Trained to exchange needs for silence and feelings for safety, she spoke not in words but through weariness, sadness, and the silence behind every "success." Vigilance calcified into a body that forgot how to breathe. Cancer wasn't the first warning—just the one I couldn't disregard.

It wasn't the symptoms I ignored—it was what they signified. My body had been whispering truths I wasn't ready to hear, so I clung to the illusion until it collapsed.

Even the most polished performances can fracture. My curated life started to splinter—hairline cracks in a world held together by sheer will. I convinced myself cancer was behind me, burying fear alongside childhood wounds and silent grief. Rather than slow down,

I doubled down—building a flawless façade I prayed would muffle the ache.

But this wasn't just about cancer; it represented the cost of a life lived in constant dis-ease, never safe enough to soften.

What began as childhood hypervigilance evolved into a sacred tremor of awakening. My body found its voice—not in screams, but in sensation, intuition, and truth.

My body was no longer a battlefield; it had become an oracle.

In the spring of 2017, just as the unraveling began, we traveled to Italy—a long-awaited trip that felt like a peculiar interlude between knowing and not knowing. Our flat near the Colosseum opened onto a sunlit courtyard filled with vibrant colors. Every morning, sunlight softened the sharp edges of my dread. One of those mornings, I paced the creaking floorboards, bracing for a call I knew would change everything.

My heart raced. My thoughts spiraled, untethered and loud. I searched for something—anything—to anchor me.

That's when I saw it: a blue morpho butterfly magnet on the fridge, its iridescent wings catching the light. Beneath it, a Chinese proverb: "Just when the caterpillar thought the world was over, it became a butterfly."

Those words didn't just catch my eye—they cut through the noise—a quiet prophecy. I realized that breaking down isn't always a dead end. Sometimes, it's the beginning of something new. The cocoon isn't a coffin; it's a gateway. Every crack and rough edge holds the potential for transformation.

The return of cancer erased all denial. It stripped me bare. It summoned the quiet pain of the child who had always carried too much. The identity I had built—of grit and performance—crumbled like old scaffolding. I stood barefoot among the rubble of my becoming. Illusions, gone.

Gill Cousteau was with me, treading water just beyond the veil, whispering:

> *"Remember who you are. You were never just a patient.*
> *You were a seeker of the deep."*

I didn't have those words then. It didn't feel like remembering—it felt like being lost at sea. I was adrift, unmoored. But now I understand: I wasn't disappearing. I was dissolving.

And then—as if the universe had waited for me to remember—the silence broke. My phone rang.

My oncologist delivered the words that every breast cancer patient dreads:

"Your cancer is back. It's metastatic—stage 4. It has spread. There is no cure."

The diagnosis struck like lightning—swift, searing, and inescapable. Time collapsed. I dropped to my knees under the weight of mortality. A storm erupted—denial, terror, sorrow, and rage—all howling through the hollow chambers of my being. I remember only one thing—echoing like a curse in the dark:

> *YOU-ARE-GOING-TO-DIE.*

The veil between life and death thinned. I stood barefoot at its edge. And then—something ancient stirred. A voice rose—not from outside, but from my marrow:

> *NOT YET, GILLIAN.*

My journey wasn't ending. The path split, calling me into the sacred unknown.

Roads are not destinations; they are invitations—shaped by intention, surrender, and spirit. Shaking and peeled open by revelation, I offered my white flag—not in defeat, but in devotion. For the first time, I listened. And the universe responded with a silence so profound that it cracked me open.

Confronting mortality shattered every illusion. The diagnosis wasn't merely clinical—it was a reckoning. I returned to the US with a prognosis of fewer than five years to live. My carefully constructed life—identity, success, and stability—began to crumble. Yet nothing cut deeper than the thought of my children reaching for a mother who was no longer present.

I felt powerless, wrecked by grief, haunted by the echo of Violet's voice telling me I had failed. The shock unmoored me—part dream, part devastation. Memories, trauma, and ego surfaced like stirred sediment, swirling into a tempest of sorrow and confusion.

Yet from the wreckage, something emerged—ancient, holy, and beyond comprehension. A cocoon formed—not of silk, but of stardust and surrender. I was suspended within it, dissolving.

My inner self no longer fit. Grief seeped through my pores. Rage pulsed. Fear buzzed in my teeth. My body felt foreign, empty, and electrified with sorrow. I melted into the mattress like wax to a flame—timeless, raw. I surrendered—not in defeat but in reverence.

What followed was silence. Then light. Then a question:

What might happen if I stopped performing strength and started embodying truth?

That was the beginning.

For four weeks, I retreated into the shadows of my bedroom. Daylight blurred into gloom. Silence hung like fog.

The blinds remained closed. Dirty dishes piled up beside an abandoned journal and a lavender candle, now lacking its scent. The air thickened with sweat, stillness, and despair. A trail of laundry—hospital gowns, robes, and children's pajamas—snaked from the bathroom to the bed.

Some mornings, I couldn't tell if it was dawn or dusk.

Kailen's small footsteps paused at the door, like a tide uncertain whether it should come in.

Once, through the thin wood, I heard him whisper, "Mama, are you asleep again?"

That question shattered me.

Not because of the words, but the innocence behind them. No judgment—only confusion. Only loss. I heard what I feared most:

Where are you, Mama? Why won't you come back?

Shame surged like a fever. I had longed to be the mother I never had—present, nurturing, and strong. But here I was, hiding in the dark while my child waited outside, unsure if I still belonged to him. I felt unworthy of his love, terrified that I was becoming a ghost in his childhood.

I wasn't just absent; I was teaching him something dangerous: that love can vanish behind closed doors, that grief can overshadow tenderness, and that pain can transform mothers into shadows.

When I started to care for myself, I learned to nurture Kailen from a place of wholeness—not hurt. I attended to the little girl inside me—the one who longed to be held, heard, and loved. I slowed down, softened, and listened—not to impress, but to understand.

Kailen reached for me with trust. He saw a mother who could cry without crumbling, who could hold his big emotions and still remain present. Our bond didn't grow from perfection; it grew from healing. When I gave myself what I had once been denied, I could finally offer it to him.

He doesn't just see a mother who survived. He feels a mother who is healing—who chooses to show up with an open heart.

But while one child observed my return, another was starting to sense the quiet outline of my absence.

I wanted to scream, *I'm still here, baby! I'm trying.* But the words dissolved before they could reach the air—undone by everything I couldn't hold.

My daughter Layke was only eight months old, cradled in the earliest season of life, while I unraveled beside her. I was present, but not entirely. Her babyhood unfolded in the shadow of my sorrow, and I feared my absence was being etched into her first memories. The burden of mothering while falling apart was almost too much to bear.

And yet, she became my golden thread—delicate yet unbreakable. In her eyes, I saw the girl I once was, reaching for the mother I was still becoming.

So, I sank deeper—not in surrender, but in shame—collapsing inward, searching for something that was still intact.

I couldn't move. The bed became my cocoon—a womb of undoing. I curled like a question mark, wrapped in gauze, grief, and everything I hadn't yet healed.

At first, it felt like death. I wasn't sure what was disintegrating faster: my body or my sense of self. Pain pooled in my hips and ribs.

Memories rose like ghosts. I spoke to my younger selves—footed-pajama girls and mascara-smudged teens—and finally told them:

"It wasn't your fault."

At night, I stared at the ceiling fan spinning like a slow-moving galaxy—time unraveling above me. I was no longer waiting to be saved. I was dissolving—cell by cell, breath by breath—into a sacred darkness that felt less like death, and more like becoming.

I didn't know what I was becoming—only that I was no longer who I had been. In that liminal stillness, I whispered prayers not for survival but for rebirth. At first, I thought I was falling apart. But in the silence, a presence began to form. I noticed the way shadows danced across the walls, how dust shimmered like glitter suspended in midair. Beyond the door, life continued—Kailen's toys clinked, Boe's footsteps echoed, and Layke's gentle coos reached out for a mother who had vanished.

These glimpses tethered me to the world I believed I had already abandoned. Somewhere between surrender and silence, I realized this wasn't just a collapse—it was the beginning of a return. Then came the shift: a golden beam of sunlight slipped through a crack in the blind and spilled across the floor.

My breath returned—not just to survive but to thrive.

The room, once a prison, was transformed into a refuge. The silence spoke. The walls embraced me like arms. The bed was no longer a confinement—it became a sanctuary.

The darkness had done its sacred work. I was listening.

I emerged not healed, but whole. Not unbroken, but reassembled.

I turned inward, into the sanctum of my soul, searching for the wisdom buried beneath the ruins of all I had lost.

I remembered: I didn't just arrive here. I drifted in on a cosmic river, a glimmer of stardust cradled in my mother's womb, sent to Earth to continue a journey etched in the language of light.

Now grounded in flesh and breath, I recognized the shattering for what it truly was—not destruction, but initiation. I needed to return to the womb-like waters, where what had hardened could soften and dissolve. Each fracture carried its own frequency, its own lesson.

As I relinquished control, each fissure began to resonate, creating a new constellation of self. I have come to trust the golden truth of kintsugi: light doesn't avoid our fractures; it seeks them.

My brokenness was never a failure. It was a gateway. I wasn't falling apart—I was breaking open. Weary to my core, I surrendered to the cloak of darkness, not out of fear, but as a rite of passage.

I no longer needed to force life into shape; I needed to loosen my grip and let the current carry me. By doing so, I released the maps I once clung to: the valleys I longed to wander, the rivers I had intended to cross, and the dreams etched on distant horizons. I allowed them all to drift away. And in that stillness, I offered myself something sacred: rest.

I listened to my breath, the ancient pulse within, and returned to the tranquil waters of my mind.

As shadows deepened, a soft light emerged. With it came grief—for the years unlived, the moments vanished, and the radiant self I had abandoned to belong to a world that couldn't see me. The weight I carried wasn't destiny—it was resistance. Only surrender could reshape the path. Only trust could return the pen to my hand.

I stopped running. I stood still and asked: "Is this anger ... or is it grief in disguise?"

Because if it were grief, rage could never free me. Only a sacred passage through could. And on the other side? Liberation. Return. Beginning. Rising.

With motherhood as the golden thread of purpose—and cancer the catalyst that cracked me open—I was ready. Despite the prophecy engraved in my bones, I chose life. With fresh eyes and a fiery spirit, I moved toward wholeness—and rose.

And then, like a tide reaching back for the shore, life called me. One tranquil morning, golden light spilled through the window. I picked up my phone for the first time in weeks. A voicemail awaited:

"Hey Gilly, it's Amy. The pool's way too quiet without your mermaid energy. We've got lanes tomorrow—come stir the waters. Bring your magic. We miss you."

Before cancer returned, I swam with a local triathlon club of warrior moms—women who carved time from chaos to flow through water, earth, and air. Hearing her voice felt like a whisper from a forgotten part of myself, urging me to return home.

With trembling courage and a heart attuned to the sacredness of every step, I said yes. Yes to movement. Yes to possibility. Yes to life.

I gave it my all to return. And by "everything," I mean standing once more on the same pool-tiled edge where I had once broken— pregnant, bald, one-breasted, and trembling with shame.

Back then, I was raw, pleading to be saved. Now, I had returned— not for rescue, but for reclamation.

I lifted the veil of isolation. Every step carried the weight of grief, anger, and memory. My limbs didn't shake from fear, but from the sacred weight of return. The pool was no longer a battlefield; it had become a baptismal font. Every step toward the water felt like resurrection.

When I plunged in, it wasn't just my body—it was every broken part I had once abandoned. Together, we submerged—not to forget, but to remember. The water embraced me like a long-lost mother. With each stroke, I surrendered worry, grief, and control. I embodied rhythm and flow.

In that sacred stillness, space expanded—and within it, I glimpsed a future not chased but embraced. Somewhere between breath and buoyancy, she returned—Gill Cousteau, the wild sea daughter I once envisioned in a windowless basement.

Born from silence and saltwater dreams, she swam beside me—not as a fantasy, but as a truth I had forgotten. The girl with gills and guts, who once escaped chaos through imagined tides, lived within me. She didn't ask me to be strong; she reminded me that I already was. I was fluid, fierce, and whole.

That swim wasn't just movement—it was a rewilding. The pool became a womb, reshaping me and teaching me to trust the current.

I no longer sought healing through control but through communion. I needed to be held by something vast, elemental, and alive.

That initial step into the university pool awakened something primal—an echo of the first waters that cradled me: first in my mother's womb, then in the Earth's.

I thought I was swimming laps. In reality, I was embarking on a journey—one that would lead me to a messenger from the deep. Someone who would recognize me long before I recognized myself.

What began in chlorinated stillness would soon be answered by the ocean's vast embrace—a deeper immersion, not only in water, but also in memory.

After my diagnosis, Boe gave me a cherished gift—not just a plane ticket, but an escape. He arranged for me to visit my dear friend

Dr. Nan Hauser at her marine biology institute on the remote island of Rarotonga. He understood that my spirit thrived near water—immersed, drifting, or simply breathing in its salty air. An ocean adventure in Rarotonga was exactly what I needed.

It was a lifeline, but even paradise couldn't protect me from what I was carrying.

Grief was raw and trembling as I moved cautiously toward the unknown. My life had been built on trauma, silence, and secrets—but I had no defenses left.

I recalled Kahlil Gibran's poem: "The river trembles before merging with the sea." I, too, had reached that edge. There was no turning back. I could no longer remain on the shoreline. I needed to leap.

It took immense courage to uncover the layers of my past—to confront the pain beneath the accolades. I stumbled, unsteady, like a newborn moose on ice, learning the awkward grace of self-compassion. Vulnerability wasn't elegant; it was messy, slippery, and full of mistakes.

But I still showed up—shaking but determined.

With compassion, I let the truth surface. I allowed myself to feel everything, without judgment. Some days, it was like being skinned alive—raw, exposed, and aching.

But this journey wasn't just about facing cancer. It was about liberating the part of me who had never been embraced—never told she didn't have to bear it all alone.

Every stroke toward the sea became a return to her: the saltwater dreamer rising not as a wound but as the wild woman I was finally becoming. She had always been present, just beneath the surface—salty and fearless. She didn't seek pain; she pursued wonder.

And when I finally listened, I realized that what I'd been searching for had never left. That brilliant, free-spirited part of me—fluid, untamed, and curious—had been waiting in the shadows. I reassembled her—not as she once was, but into something sacred and whole. My light shone not in spite of the cracks, but because of them.

And it was in the ocean—my first sanctuary, my eternal mirror—that she stirred most vividly. The ocean's fluidity, kaleidoscope of color, and ancient rhythm awakened something long buried within me. In her embrace, I softened, and Gill Cousteau came to life.

It now feels inevitable that I have become a marine biologist. My love for the sea wasn't learned—it was remembered. When I was seven and saw Dr. Sylvia Earle in *National Geographic*, something within me ignited. Sylvia was wild, wise, and unafraid. In her, I found freedom to live with purpose.

The ocean wasn't merely my passion; it was my way home.

That path led me to Rarotonga—a volcanic jewel in the South Pacific, lush and pristine, shimmering like a dream made real—where I would volunteer my expertise to help Nan with whale research.

Surrounded by coral reefs and the warm waters where humpback whales give birth, Rarotonga is a place where the sacred and the unseen coexist—where vibrant reefs yield to the mysteries of the deep.

The humpbacks travel thousands of kilometers from Antarctica to these waters—not to escape, but to create. Their courtship is breathtaking, revealing something ancient and familiar: the sovereignty of the feminine, the wisdom of instinct, and the power of choice. I was also drawn to these waters—not just to witness the sacred but to remember I belonged to it.

That recognition stirred something profound. As the whales returned to their ancestral waters, I felt a call back to my own.

My childhood alter ego Gill Cousteau was no longer a figment of my imagination. As a marine biologist, I once dove for data. But this time, I arrived in Rarotonga to dive for something more profound—not answers, but reunion. I was searching for myself—not the scientist, not the patient, nor the mother—but the soul that still believed something sacred awaited beneath the surface.

Fearless, bold, and wild like the sea, I plunged into her tranquil waters, giddy with anticipation. Light refracted around me like a blessing. Weightless, I floated—cradled like a newborn, spinning through somersaults.

For a moment, I forgot I was dying.

Like a dream, I encountered my past selves again—the girl in the basement, the dreamer, the swimmer—and embraced all of them. The sea didn't just welcome me; she remembered me.

And then, as if by magic, *she* arrived.

Out of the silence, *Kanikani iti*—"Tiny Dancer" in Māori—arose from the deep. A newborn humpback whale, accompanied by her massive mother, emerged.

They didn't just appear. They summoned.

As I moved, Kanikani iti followed in sync, pausing as if she sensed I needed to be seen. When our foreheads aligned, I saw myself—complete. A memory, a return.

Her mother lingered nearby—watchful, trusting, and serene—a matriarchal sentinel anchoring our communion.

My heart swelled with reverence.

At that moment, I encountered the divine—not in doctrine, but in its essence. Not in temples crafted by hands, but in the vastness that encompasses everything. It resided in the stillness, in the silence between us, and most profoundly—in the whale's eye. That gaze penetrated every layer of illusion. It didn't just see me—it remembered me. The ocean became my cathedral. The whales, my messengers of what had always been sacred.

The Māori consider whales as ancestors, divine carriers of transformation and guardians of the spirit. In their presence, I felt alive—not as a diagnosis, but as a soul in sacred motion. They reminded me that

I am not defined by what brought me to my knees, but by how I rise after falling.

In the months leading up to that encounter, I had been shedding versions of myself built on survival and silence. Now, suspended in sacred blue, I wasn't unraveling—I was reforming. Maybe not with wings, but with fins.

I came to the ocean to escape death. But it wasn't death that met me; it was the divine—quiet, breathless, and vast.

In the eye of the whale, I saw the truth: I was not lost. I was being returned.

That moment didn't cure me; it brought me back to myself.

In Kanikani iti's gaze, I wasn't a body in decline on the precipice of death. I wasn't diagnosed with breast cancer. I was a wild soul—wandering, sacred, and remembered—I was Gill Cousteau.

When the Earth Quakes, the Mountains Rise

Seven years had passed since I first heard the words that fractured my world: "incurable metastatic breast cancer."

During that time, life unfolded in ways I could never have scripted—shaped by sorrow, strength, transformation, and sacred return.

Layke, who was just eight months old when I was diagnosed, was now eight—curious, wild, and ocean-hearted.

Kailen, the child who had once whispered behind a bedroom door, had grown into the quiet strength of a confident boy raised in the shadow of his mother's becoming.

On a perfect evening off the coast of Costa Rica, Layke and I stood barefoot at the edge of a catamaran, the Pacific Ocean shimmering below.

The sun hung low—an amber orb slipping into the sea.

We were breathless, hands clasped in electric anticipation.

I gazed into her wide brown eyes—still filled with wonder, now softened by the quiet strength of a girl shaped by her mother's rebirth.

In that moment, I wasn't just her teacher; I was a witness to her growth, her radiance, and her truth.

The countdown started: *three, two, one—*

And together, we surrendered to the sky.

We leaped, laughed, and surfaced anew. Saltwater mixed with sunlight.

Breathless and glowing, we climbed back aboard—just as the final golden thread of the day slipped beneath the sea.

And then, something extraordinary emerged from beneath the surface.

With slow, ceremonial grace, the tail of a humpback whale arched upward toward the heavens . . .

—It was *her*.

The messenger. The mirror. The memory.

Her reappearance wasn't a coincidence. It was choreography.

A benediction.

I stood at the rail, salt drying on my skin, hair clinging to my shoulders, and wept—not out of grief, but out of reverence.

In that moment, every thread of my becoming—mother, survivor, seeker, and soul—was woven into a luminous whole.

Even the child I once hid—the one exiled to the basement, silenced by shame, and comforted only by saltwater dreams—stood beside me. Not merely as a ghost of trauma but as a golden thread woven into the tapestry of my wholeness.

The ocean had held me in dissolution. The whale had returned me to remembrance. And now, I felt the mountains within me begin to rise. This journey was never just about yielding; it was also about ascending. When the Earth quakes, mountains do not retreat—they rise. And I, too, had risen—from silence, trauma, and surrender.

Mountains, like whales, are more than metaphors—they are mirrors. The sea taught me to trust my wildness. The mountains taught me to meet myself at the summit—not to conquer, but to witness my truth. Their stillness reminds me that transformation doesn't always whisper; sometimes it quakes. Each climb quiets the noise and reconnects me to what truly matters. I've learned that surrender is not collapse—it is power in another form.

The mountain was never a destination; it was a return. I didn't climb to overcome. I ascended to remember. Each step was not an ending but a sacred convergence with the part of me that had always known the way.

And I didn't rise alone. I rose for them—for the little boy who once whispered behind a door, uncertain if his mama would return. For the baby girl who cried out in the dark, needing comfort, a lullaby, and an embrace. They are the heartbeat of my life and the spark that fuels my becoming. Every step I've taken toward healing is also a step toward the mother I longed to be—not perfect, but present. Not untouched by pain, but transformed by it.

Gill Cousteau wasn't just a dream; she embodied the wild, saltwater part of me—the fearless self who dove into the depths where I once drowned. I didn't create her to escape; I summoned her forward to survive. But over time, she became something more: not a fantasy, but a reflection of my essence waiting to be remembered.

She had been my sanctuary for years—a saltwater whisper through grief, healing, and awakening. Eventually, the boundary between us dissolved. I didn't need to become her; I realized I had always been her. She wasn't a mask; she was a memory. The girl who imagined Gill Cousteau rescuing her had become the woman who could rescue herself.

Through oceans, diagnoses, and darkness, we were never apart. We were always one.

I now carry her into the heart of my daily life. As the founder of the iRise Above Foundation, I don't lead with spreadsheets or forecasts—I lead from instinct. A wild, knowing current flows through me—a river of intuition shaped by the tides and tremors of life. I listen to what stirs beneath the surface and trust what rises. I lead with a backbone forged in saltwater and surrender.

This wildness—the same essence that danced with whales and wept on mountaintops—guides how I raise my children, how I show up in the world, and how I heal. iRise Above was born not from certainty, but from stillness. In the aftermath of my diagnosis, I recognized myself in other young women—daughters, mothers, seekers—searching for meaning in the rubble. I didn't create iRise Above to help them merely survive. I created it to help them thrive.

It became a sanctuary where healing isn't rushed, where stories are sacred, and no woman rises alone.

I did not leave my past behind—I transformed it. The girl who learned to disappear so others could shine now stands fully in her light. My healing was not only from cancer, but from the silence that shaped me. Every stroke in the sea and every surrender on the mountain was for her—for the girl who believed she had to carry it all.

I didn't just survive—I rewrote the story. I became the voice, the mother, and the truth-bearer I always needed.

I am a woman who remembers. I am the one who rises. This is not an ending—

It is the tide turning.

A breath, returned.

A truth, rekindled.

Becoming never ends.

Gill Cousteau lives on—not in the sea, but in every breath I take, every wave I encounter, and every woman I rise beside. She is not a memory—she is the alchemist within, transforming salt into gold, pain into offering, and shadow into song. She encapsulates the saltwater truth of who I've always been. Now, she swims in every sacred rising—not just remembered, but reborn.

AUTHOR BIO

Gillian Lichota is the founder and CEO of the iRise Above Foundation and the visionary lead author of *Rising Above: Our Transformational Journey to Wholeness After Breast Cancer*. As a mother, marine biologist, sacred space-holder, and truth-teller, Gillian creates environments where young women can transform pain into power and embrace their fullest expression.

At thirty-four, while pregnant with her first child, Gillian was diagnosed with breast cancer—a rupture that collided joy with mortality and forever altered the landscape of her life. Years later, after the birth of her second child, the cancer returned—this time metastatic and terminal. Her prognosis was grim. But Gillian did not collapse; she cracked open.

From that sacred fracture, the iRise Above Foundation emerged.

Founded in 2017, iRise Above is more than a nonprofit; it is a living sanctuary for transformation. Under Gillian's leadership, the foundation empowers young women diagnosed with breast cancer to reclaim their voice, agency, and wholeness. Through evidence-based tools, integrative healing practices, and soul-rooted sisterhood, iRise Above guides women not only to survive but also to thrive—body, mind, and spirit.

Before her diagnosis, Gillian spent two decades as a marine biologist, exploring Arctic ecosystems and global change. Her scientific journey mirrored her spiritual one: immersion, depth, and reverence for life in all its wild forms. Today, she channels that same devotion into the soul's terrain—guiding others through inner oceans of grief, rebirth, and self-reclamation.

Her writing serves as both a map and a mirror—lyrical, raw, and infused with truth. In her lead chapter "The Alchemy of Becoming," Gillian invites readers to witness what happens when we stop hiding our scars and instead gild them with gold. The *Rising Above* anthology is not merely a collection of survival stories—it is a constellation of origin stories, where each woman's truth shines like a kintsugi seam: broken, reassembled, and made radiant through the act of becoming.

Originally from Canada, Gillian continues to scale both physical and metaphorical mountains. She draws strength from untamed landscapes and deep surrender, returning time and again to the sacred truth: Rising isn't about returning to who we were, but evolving into who we were always meant to be.

You can follow Gillian's journey and learn more about the iRise Above Foundation at www.iriseabovefoundation.org, on Instagram @iRise_Above and @gillian.lichota, Facebook @IRiseAboveFoundation, YouTube @iRiseAboveFoundation, or by contacting her at glichota@iriseabovefoundation.org.

APRIL STEARNS

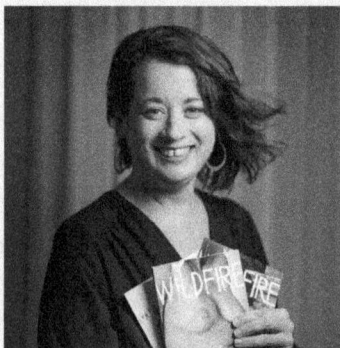

I had believed the mother-daughter bond was always one bad moment away from breaking. But now I see it differently: when it's built with presence and care, it can bend, stretch—even through cancer—and not break.

FORGED
IN THE FIRE

On Illness, Motherhood, and Becoming a
First-Generation Cycle Breaker

The first time my daughter looks at me like I am a stranger is the day I come home without a breast.

It's a warm September evening in 2012. I'm sitting in the only sliver of shade near the hot tub, too tired to do anything but exist. My eyes are ringed with exhaustion, my body a strange, bandaged version of what it was just yesterday. Across from me, my four-year-old floats silent and still, her nose pressed to the side of the tub, her brown eyes locked on mine. She doesn't splash. She doesn't smile. She stares, unmoving, like she's trying to understand what happened to the mother she knew.

We are so fucked.

* * *

Twenty-four hours earlier, my daughter and I spent our first night apart as my left breast was amputated.

When I returned home from the hospital, I was relieved to see my little Nia. I expected her to be bright and happy. Instead, she barely looked at me. Seeing her pull back, I realized I wasn't just changed—I was unrecognizable to her. Maybe even to me. I was noticeably weaker than when she left me, now bandaged and drained, with tubes containing mysterious red and pink fluid protruding from my chest.

After her initial hesitation, she suddenly wanted to jump into my arms, but now it was my turn to be cautious. My husband Joe, always the protector, stepped between us and lifted her, gently reminding her to be careful with me. She buried her face in his chest and cried.

"I want you to have another surgery," she wailed at me. "I want you to have a new boob!"

My heart broke as I realized my mistake. I had removed only the breast with the tumor and had no plans for reconstruction. That wasn't the mistake, though. The mistake was assuming she wouldn't need a story to hold onto. I left her with absence, not explanation.

A crack is opening in our mother-daughter bond. I've seen what happens when illness swallows a mother whole—and deep down, I'm terrified it is happening again. *We are so fucked.*

* * *

My sister-in-law Whitney arrives like her own version of Mary Poppins on the summer breeze. Beautiful, six-foot, brunette, in through the door, sweet relief washes over us in the form of her cheery disposition and a duffel bag filled with distracting games and stickers.

My brother's wife is a dynamic, full-of-energy, twenty-five-year-old; a one-woman rescue squad, delivering us from the dark, moody, postsurgical trauma fog. I adore her. As she enters, Joe, Nia, and I collectively exhale. We all know Whitney will help Nia feel better.

Despite that, a prickle of cold anxiety creeps into my chest, curling into the space where my breast once was, as if the loss has left a door ajar for my worst nightmare to wedge its way through. Nia's anger jolts me because I recognize it. I know how it feels to be the child left hurting by a mother pulled away by something happening to her body.

Bald, weak, and half-mutilated, I need Whitney here. I am the one who begged her to come all the way from Montana. But as I look at her now, my breath catches. She excels in every place I lack: energy, ease, wholeness. She's everything I'm not. And what if Nia sees it? What if she chooses light over the shadow I feel I'm becoming in illness?

"Where do you want to sleep tonight, Bug?" Whitney asks, catching my leaping daughter in her arms.

"With you!" Nia squeals.

I swallow a lump in my throat. Honestly, I had hoped Nia would sleep with Whitney so I wouldn't worry about jabs to my surgical site in the night. The chance to rest undisturbed is a relief. But still, Nia's preference for her flawless young aunt feels like a rejection. Maybe she doesn't need me anymore. Has our bond been amputated too?

We have just seven days before Whitney flies back to Montana. *We are so fucked.*

Six Months Earlier

It's a dark February night. The house is quiet and I'm nursing Nia to sleep in the living room. Joe is already in bed, and our skittish black cat, sensing the littlest, most unpredictable human in the family is contained, has emerged to bathe herself. I love this time of night. Usually, I nurse Nia to sleep in our bed, but tonight, we're cuddled on the couch so I can binge a little more *Orange Is the New Black*.

At nearly four, Nia and I have had a beautiful, longer-than-most breastfeeding relationship. It didn't come easily—my inverted nipples made the early weeks excruciating—but when it finally became effortless, I wasn't in a hurry to let it go. Besides, nursing calmed the larger-than-life emotions of my "threenager."

Lately, though, Nia seems frustrated with my left breast, nursing for a moment, then unlatching to switch sides. I don't think much of it. As a toddler, she's mostly nursing for comfort. She tries again. Her mouth finds the nipple, but something in her pulls back. Restless, she switches again. It's as if her body already knows what mine hasn't yet discovered. I admire her long lashes as her eyes finally close into milk-drunk sleep. Absent-mindedly, I massage the top of my left breast to coax the milk down. That's when I feel it. My fingers land on something that doesn't belong.

A hands-width from my armpit, where chest slopes into breast, there is an unmistakable golf-ball-sized lump. Once I feel it, I can't stop. I prod, I press. I already know.

As soon as Nia is asleep, I carry her to our bed and turn to Joe.

"Can you feel something for me?" I ask, heart pounding, finger stroking the spot.

He throws back the comforter, tossing his phone aside. Wordlessly, he puts his hand where I indicate. He prods the lump, staring into my eyes.

Finally, he says, "What the hell is that?!"

That night, I keep one hand on my chest and the other wrapped around Nia. The fear pushing ice water through my veins isn't just about what the lump means for me; it's about what it might take from her.

We are so fucked.

* * *

Within a few short weeks, I've had the lump palpated by my gynecologist, experienced my first mammogram, received a breast ultrasound by a tight-lipped technician whose lack of warmth filled me with anxiety, and celebrated my thirty-fifth birthday with a week in Lake Tahoe. Watching my child play in the snow, I couldn't help but wonder if it would be my last birthday.

Now I'm lying face down on an elevated gurney, my breasts hanging through two holes cut out, one for each pendulum, while a doctor performs a needle core biopsy on the lump. They've numbed the area, but the sound cuts through everything. *Ka-chunk! Ka-chunk!* Like an industrial stapler firing into flesh. After each *ka-chunk!*, the doctor deposits little cylinders of breast tissue into a petri dish held by a nurse. I can't see the doctor, and I try not to imagine my disembodied breasts dangling in front of his face.

Beside me, I can make out the nurse holding a petri dish, if I look out the side of my left eye. As the doctor deposits each fleshy piece from the "stapler" to the dish, she fiddles with the contents, moving some of it with her long tweezers to another dish. Watching her work makes me feel nauseous. I move my focus away from her hands and settle my gaze on her head instead. I'm surprised to see she is about my age. Her long, black, curly hair stands out against her turquoise scrubs. *It suits her*, I think.

"How old is your daughter?" she asks, catching my eye. I realize that she noticed I was looking at her.

I smile, despite having been caught staring. Happy for the distraction, I answer, "She's almost four."

"Oh my god, I'm so sorry. She's so young," she says, her eyes wide, filled with an emotion I can't quite identify.

I'm confused.

"If you need someone to watch her, I can," she goes on.

"Okay . . . thank you . . . ?" *Why would someone need to watch her,* I wonder.

I don't know what to say. I close my eyes as my mind starts to skitter around my brain like a cornered animal.

Why will I need a stranger to watch my daughter? The question pings in my brain again like an urgent alarm going off. There is something here I need to pay close attention to, but I don't know what.

The silence stretches, punctuated by the *ka-chunk!* of the biopsy tool.

Suddenly, I register another sound in the room: sniffling. My eyes slide back to the nurse's face, and what I see chills me to my core. She is crying. She is crying for me and my daughter, understanding something I don't yet.

We are so fucked.

* * *

In the days following the biopsy, I meet my oncology team and receive the diagnosis: I have breast cancer. The tumor is large—about seven centimeters—and classified as Stage 3c, which means it's advanced and has spread to my lymph nodes. The specific type is called HER2-positive invasive ductal carcinoma, a rapidly growing cancer driven by a protein that causes the cells to multiply quickly. I don't yet understand what any of it really means, only that it sounds urgent. *Serious.* Like something that won't let me return to life as I knew it.

Treatment is set to begin in three weeks, starting with chemotherapy, followed by a mastectomy, and thirty-five rounds of radiation. The final layer in this treatment plan is thirteen months of biotherapy with the drug Herceptin. I learn that, unlike chemotherapy, which attacks all fast-growing cells in the body, cancer, nails, hair, etc., biotherapy drugs specifically look for and target cancer cells in the body. In my case, the HER2 receptors of my breast cancer type.

"I hope to have you done with the big stuff by Christmas," Dr. Yen, my thirty-something, cheerful-but-no-nonsense chemo oncologist, tells me the first time we meet, referring to the gauntlet of chemo, surgery, and radiation I've got ahead of me.

Christmas? It's March. I start to do the mental math. *That's nine months away!*

The longest illness I'd had before this was mono when I was a senior in college—a month of bone-crushing fatigue I tried to ignore. I kept up a full course load, worked nights, all while telling myself I was just tired. I didn't know how to stop without free-falling off the cliff I watched my mother succumb to with her illness. No one in my family had modeled healthy rest and recuperation. With cancer, I hit the same wall—but this time, there's no pushing through. The stakes are higher. For the first time in my life, I have to learn it is safe for me to be sick. More than that, because of my daughter, I have to learn that I can surrender to healing without losing myself to the illness.

It is difficult to comprehend the magnitude of the path ahead of me for many reasons, including the paradoxical reality of the whirlwind weeks of diagnosis during which doctors kept saying variations of, "You're so healthy; other than the cancer, I mean."

Translation: *You're so young.*

Before the prescribed five months of chemotherapy could begin, I needed to complete a series of scans using contrast dye to determine if breast cancer cells were stealthily spreading to other parts of my body. "Breast cancer," Dr. Yen said, "has a proclivity for setting up shop in the liver, lungs, bones, and brain." Not knowing exactly what these scans will mean for breastfeeding my daughter, I call my local breastfeeding support person at the La Leche League organization. Tearfully, I explain the devastating situation, and she, sadly and gently, confirms that the use of contrast dye in the scans is unsafe for Nia to ingest through my breast milk. With no supply of frozen pumped milk to use, I must wean Nia today, right now, before tomorrow's MRI.

Everything about this timeline is jarring. When I started down the path of breastfeeding, I didn't know how long we would do it. I had wanted to go for at least two years, if possible. As the months and then years slipped by and breastfeeding became part of our routine, I learned about and loved the idea of child-led weaning. Child-led weaning would be entirely on Nia's terms: She would stop when it no longer served her. I had already agonized over and ultimately quit a job that wasn't supportive of breastfeeding early on in my parenting journey. Here it was again: the outside world telling me I must wean. Not sometime soon. Not next week. Right now.

The thought hits me like a tidal wave: What if cancer is going to take not just my breast, but the version of motherhood I fought so hard to build? Later, I learn all the ways cancer is a thief; the end of breastfeeding is the first of many cruel losses. The hormonal crash that follows weaning feels like the floor falling out. The physical separation between us is abrupt. Before cancer, we were always together—an attachment-parenting family.

How do we stay close when my body is forcing us apart? Will my child reject me if I cannot breastfeed her? Will cancer confirm my deepest fear that I am not fit to be a mother, turning me into a version of my mother?

I hear my mother's sneering voice resounding in my head: "April rejected my breast. She rejected *me*."

This isn't just about milk. It's about the distance that wasn't there yesterday but is now forcing us apart. It's the beginning of everything breaking.

* * *

My name was one of the best things I ever got from my dad.

Growing up, people always said, "I know when your birthday is!" with a wink.

But they didn't know because while my parents expected me on April Fools' Day 1977, I was born a month premature in early March.

"Why didn't they name you 'March' then?" was the frequent retort.

"Too militant," I learned to deadpan.

See, I can joke too.

My parents were Martin and Ingrid. Ingrid graduated from high school six months early so they could marry within a month of her eighteenth birthday. She was eager to escape her parents and start adult life. Martin, four years her senior and best friends with her older brother, had departed for college in Wyoming but returned to California, and Ingrid, soon after. He was the spitting image of Frank Zappa: tall and slim with olive skin, dark eyes, black hair, and a signature handlebar mustache that he only shaved a couple of times in my life. Ingrid was his opposite in almost every way: petite with curls shot through with gold, perfectly framing her sparkling green eyes.

She was fiery, assertive, and uncompromising, whereas he was patient, soft-spoken, and gentle.

Two years after their wedding, I was born. The day they brought me home from the hospital, it was finally the month of my namesake, April, and it was snowing big, fluffy flakes, unusual for spring in the Santa Cruz Mountains. At 3500 feet above sea level, the mountains were thick with towering Douglas Fir and coastal redwoods, forming a barrier between the still orchard-dotted Silicon Valley of the late 1970s and the Pacific Ocean.

My parents carried me into their tiny wood-sided cabin and placed my five-pound body in a cradle before the large stone fireplace that heated the cabin.

My premature birth required me to stay in the neonatal intensive care unit for three weeks while my lungs developed and my body cleared jaundice. My mom was discharged soon after my birth. Later, as our relationship grew increasingly strained, I would cry to my dad that she didn't love me.

He once said of the weeks I spent without her in the hospital: "She visited you that one time . . ."

By the time I was discharged, I was thriving via formula. When my brothers Dale and Kyle came into the picture years later, both carrying full-term, Ingrid became passionate about breastfeeding and joined her local La Leche League chapter. As I grew up and each year of our relationship became more strained, she would often bring up the fact that I was her only child who was not breastfed.

"You rejected me from the beginning" was something Ingrid said often when I was a teen and doing what teenagers do: starting to pull away from family life. Her green eyes would flash with anger and accusation, as if it were my fault.

It wasn't until my twenties that I learned my mom wasn't just mean, she had borderline personality disorder. Reading *Understanding the Borderline Mother* by Christine Lawson, and from there finding the Craigslist discussion board for children of borderline mothers, was the start of my healing. Suddenly, I found a way to understand and articulate my experience that others could comprehend.

In her book, Lawson describes four subtypes of mothers with borderline personality disorder (BPD): the Waif (helpless), the Hermit (fearful/avoidant), the Queen (narcissistic and controlling), and the Witch (sadistic).

My mom was a Queen/Witch.

It's hard to describe the relief of seeing the chaos I lived through described in black and white in a book. I wasn't just imagining the wickedness. It was real, and it had a psychological profile. Through my research, I came to understand that Witches want power and control over others to ensure they will not be abandoned. This is their biggest fear, and when that fear is triggered, they can become brutal and full of rage, punishing and hurting their spouses and children.

I learned young that it was best to comply. Martin, Dale, Kyle, and I entered an unspoken "Nobody rock the boat!" pact. My siblings and I lived in absolute fear of emotional, physical, and sexual violence. A war was waging within Ingrid that we could not possibly understand, but for which we were collateral damage.

As I grew up, Ingrid cast me as the "all bad kid." Everything she hated about herself, she projected onto me. Every trigger, every flaw, she saw in me. As my body developed into that of a woman, she saw me as a threat to her marriage. After I cut contact with her, I received emails from her therapists demanding, on Ingrid's behalf, that I cease an imagined sexual relationship with Martin, my father.

Ingrid always told me that a mother could not be friends with her daughter. She hated the parenting trend toward this and often mocked my friends' parents as naive. She also instilled in me a belief that everything I loved could be taken at a moment's notice. I spent the majority of my teen years grounded. If I expressed any interest in anything (my horse, my boyfriend, a TV show), it became the thing I was grounded from next.

I learned not to want things and to hold what I had loosely.

When cancer came, it fed right into my world view that I would lose what I held most dear now: my relationship with my child.

I should never have let the universe know I cared about something.

*   *   *

The week after my mastectomy, I stay in bed. From my bedroom, I listen to Nia and Whitney move through the days together, playing, cooking, and roughhousing. All day, Nia avoids me. All night, she sleeps beside her aunt.

Slowly, it occurs to me that Nia is grieving too. She has every right. The situation is quite clear to her: my breasts were *hers*. She had fed and found comfort in them daily from birth until I found the lump. I didn't put it together until now, and the realization hits me like a punch in the stomach. She thought we would resume nursing when the "big medicine" was over. In her mind, weaning was always temporary. A pause, not an end.

Maybe I knew this on some level, but I didn't want to add insult to her injury. So I avoided explaining what cancer treatment really meant. We were on a new road with no map, no GPS, and no flashlight. All through those long chemo weeks, in lieu of the comfort she received from nursing, she snuggled close and rested her head on my chest, listening to my heartbeat below the soft surface, waiting. For five and a half long months, she waited. But not only had she not been invited to resume nursing once the chemotherapy was complete, I had actually gone and done an unspeakable thing: I had a breast physically removed from my body.

Her breast was cut from my body and discarded.

And while I was relieved to have it and the cancer it had harbored gone, she was in deep mourning. Thanks to stitches and drains, my chest couldn't provide any maternal comfort when she needed it most.

We shed our tears separately, grieving the same wound in different languages. Could we somehow find our way back to each other before Whitney leaves?

* * *

On the same day my mother is buried, my best friend gives birth.

Later, I tell people I left my role at her bedside as a birth doula to attend a funeral, liking the drama of it—birth and death in a single afternoon. What I don't say is that I fled the church for the comfort of welcoming new life, running from a service for a woman I didn't recognize. In fleeing, I didn't yet understand how angry I was, or that my anger was the story I kept trying to press into the hands of others.

Inside the church, I sit in the front pew between my husband and brothers, watching my father, stooped and grief-stricken, a man who has lost his lifelong tether. *If they were a kite and string,* I think, *she would be the kite . . . now the kite is gone.* The church is packed: friends, neighbors, coworkers, all gathered to mourn a woman they thought they knew.

The service unfolds like a theater centered around a single photo. Framed by blue irises and white roses, the portrait of Ingrid showcases her perfectly styled appearance: her signature teal mascara and familiar mauve lipstick are broadcast on a grand scale. Her curated image is still doing its work, even now.

When the pastor opens the floor, a parade of strangers speaks of her kindness, her devotion, her selflessness. "She was a good mom. She was a good mom. She was a good mom." Their words beat against me like a drum, building a version of her that erases everything I endured. The rages, the control, the stringent Dial soap scraped across my tongue. No one talks about that. No one saw it.

Now I understand the funeral wasn't a reckoning. It was the telling of a story about the Ingrid they were allowed to see. She had cloaked me in invisibility to let a version of herself shine, and that day, I absorbed it all.

Years later, in the haze of cancer, I would think about the funeral again—the neat story laid over a woman whose chaos had shaped my childhood. I'd realize how easily illness, be it mental or physical, invites mythology. People want the version they can live with: the brave one, the grateful one, the redeemed one. I had seen it happen with Ingrid. I knew now how easily it could happen to me.

As I sat in that pew attending my mother's funeral just days after my wedding, I was sure of one thing.

If Ingrid fits the story of a good mom, I don't want to be a mom then.

* * *

It is now a few days after Ingrid's funeral.

Martin, Dale, Kyle, and I are squeezed into Martin's small SUV. We ride silently, our bodies tilting in unison with every tree-lined curve.

I feel a clawing desperation to escape the car, nausea creeping up from my stomach to lodge thickly in my throat. It isn't the mountain roads that make me sick. It is our destination; we are on our way to our first-ever family therapy experience: a bereavement group for people who have lost a family member.

Going was my idea. Empowered by my discovery of talk therapy, and with it, the wild relief of diagnosis (*You mean it isn't my fault? There's a name for what she has?*), I appointed myself family savior upon her death. I would guide us from the darkness of the last decades into the light with gritted teeth determination. In the previous two weeks since Ingrid died, some days being the self-appointed Suicide Aftermath Tour Guide means finally, really talking to each other about what we've endured. Today, it means letting fellow travelers in grief and loss see us in our suffering and, hopefully, show us a way out.

But I want to turn the car around. In addition to "Nobody rock the boat," our other family motto has always been "What happens in the family stays in the family."

We arrive late to the support group. As we file into the light blue linoleum-floored community center, the circle of chairs in the middle of the room is already full. Someone is talking, but stops as soon as we enter. The whole circle swivels their heads toward us. More chairs are found and added to the circle. Once we sit, the group resumes, and I feel exposed. I long for a pillow to pull into my lap, some way to place a barrier between me and the grief-stricken. I cross and uncross my arms.

Eventually, we are invited to share why we are here, starting with Martin.

"I, we, lost—" my dad struggles to get the words out, his eyes red-rimmed. He clears his throat and says hoarsely, "—my wife."

There is a pause as the group waits for more. A murmur of understanding ripples around the circle when he says nothing else. I glance around and notice the group is primarily women, mostly my grandmother's age. The one sitting beside me has a tightly-curled, tidy short 'do. Her white purse sits primly on her tan slacked lap, her Keds crossed neatly. She catches my eye and offers a kind, closed-mouth smile. My body relaxes a little. Maybe this will be okay.

Next, my youngest brother speaks. His denim-clad legs are relaxed, one foot resting on his knee. He leans back in his chair comfortably, just a person at any social gathering. He looks around the group, making eye contact. I imagine he's mentally checking off public speaking to-dos. "I'm Kyle. He's my dad," he says, indicating Martin, who is now studying his hands in his lap. "Our mom just died."

Another pregnant pause from the group, and then a murmured exhale of "Welcome, Kyle."

The invisible microphone is passed to Dale.

"Yeah, um, same," is all he mutters. His arms stay crossed tightly. He stares at the rectangular box of Kleenex in the center of the floor, a small sun in the orbiting circle of bereaved.

And now it's my turn.

"Hi, I'm April. Like they said, we lost our mom a couple of weeks ago."

I take a breath and continue, "She died by suicide. A gunshot."

There is a collective gasp.

I push on. "We're here because . . . it's hard. I'm sad but also angry? She was challenging . . . I feel abandoned, and relieved? And sad," I say.

The sob I've been holding back since my dad first spoke takes over, and no more words come out.

To my left, Dale leans forward, retrieves a tissue from the box on the floor, and hands it to me. Grateful, I dab at my mascaraed eyes, hiding briefly behind the soft white paper barrier as another murmur of welcome washes over the group.

The woman in tan slacks to my right touches my shoulder. Sniffling and wet, I turn toward her. Her baby-blue eyes pierce mine, and her hand becomes a claw, gripping my shoulder.

"Oh, honey," she says. "It's going to be okay. I lost my mom, too, years ago."

She continues, "The beautiful thing is, one day you'll open your mouth and your mom's voice will come out like she's right there with you."

I find myself speechless.

Did she not hear anything I said? How could she think that would be comforting?

What I didn't know then was that I was never in danger of merely echoing my mother's hurtful voice. The real threat was echoing her relationship to illness. With cancer looming just five years away, that was the real legacy lying in wait: wielding illness the way she did, turning it into both fortress and blade, cutting off her daughter at every attempt at love and connection.

In that moment, in the support group to which we never returned, it felt inevitable. The cycle will not be broken: I will become her.

I am so fucked.

* * *

Six months have passed since my mother's death. It's New Year's Day 2007, and Joe and I are walking around downtown Santa Cruz. Most of the boutique shops that give the town its character are closed, but the weather is mild, so the sidewalks are bustling with families looking for something to do on a sleepy holiday. Joe and I walk hand in hand, stopping to admire the jewelry in the large picture window of the antique shop where we selected our vintage wedding rings just a few months ago. Mine is a blue star sapphire set in white gold, while his is a thick band of rose gold.

I'm on the verge of my thirtieth birthday and feel brand-new in the world. There is a lightness I have never experienced before, now that Ingrid is gone. It's even more profound than when I left for college, or when, at twenty-eight, I finally stood up to her and cut contact eighteen months before her suicide. The old family mantra—what happens in the family, stays in the family—died with her. Along with it died the silence I'd carried like a second skin. I'm finding my voice, shedding the shame that clung to me, and finding solace in witnesses to what I endured.

And I am slowly rebuilding my relationship with my dad.

"I call my dad Martin now," I said to a friend over coffee when she asked how life was after the suicide.

"Oh, where did Martin come from?" she asked.

I'm confused. "What do you mean? Why did his parents name him Martin?"

"Ha!" she laughs. "No, I thought you gave him a whole new name."

Calling my mom "Ingrid" marked my need for distance. Calling my dad "Martin" came from something more profound: a realization that he had never really been a father to me. Although he was the better of my two parents, he rarely acted as a dad should. He had a history of disappearing or throwing me under the bus to stay on Ingrid's good side.

"But I did that too," I said to my therapist.

"The difference was," she replied, "he was supposed to be the adult. You were a child."

It is hard to hear. I had always cast him as a fellow victim in the family, just as tormented by Ingrid's moods and violence as we kids. Now, I was learning that he should have acted differently. He should have protected me. Calling him Martin signals a new chapter in our relationship. We will face the past and chart a new, healthy way forward.

I thought that was the hard part—facing the pain, naming it, beginning again. But years later, when cancer arrives, I realize healing is never a straight line. I pulled away from Ingrid's legacy with everything I had, but illness has a way of testing our distance from the past. It whispers: *Are you sure you've escaped? Are you sure you're not her?*

For the first time in my life, I have Martin's attention. I am no longer competing with Ingrid's rage and jealousy or his vanishing into his work. He is becoming a parent to me before my eyes. I demand that he witness my childhood pain by dragging him with me to therapy several times, during which I mostly cry and recount all the ways in which Ingrid hurt me, and he did nothing.

I share about the time at sixteen when Ingrid berated me for kissing a boy. She yelled that I was a slut who was going to get pregnant—maybe was even already pregnant. Martin sat on the couch a few feet away, silently reading the newspaper.

"Are you pregnant?!" Ingrid seethed. The rage in her eyes was terrifying, and I went from confident that one could not get pregnant from simply kissing to unsure.

"I . . . don't know."

I looked to my dad for help. Our eyes met above the edge of the newspaper, his full of sorrow, mine full of fear.

He held my gaze for a moment.

Then, wordlessly, he raised the paper and disappeared behind it.

I always thought Ingrid was between us, preventing him from being my dad. In therapy, I learned that his codependence was what was always between us.

"How does he feel about you calling him by his first name?" my friend asked.

"It doesn't matter to me how he feels about it," I said. "I am just glad we have the opportunity for him to become my Martin."

* * *

As Joe and I continue to wander down the January sidewalk, our entwined hands swinging between us, we fall in step behind a small, three-person family. The parents look to be about our age. A young girl is perched on the man's shoulders. Joe and I silently watch them as we walk. The mom is holding a pink child's cup. Every so often, she retrieves an orange Goldfish cracker from the cup and hands it up to the child. When she isn't carefully guiding a cracker into her mouth, the child has her pudgy hands on each of her dad's cheeks. The tenderness with which she holds her dad's face and his ease with her touch sends an unfamiliar jolt through my body.

I never expected to become a mother. I was scared of becoming Ingrid—or worse, giving birth to a child that embodied her rage—and I didn't know how to protect a child from the kind of mother I'd had, or from me if I became her. If no one had been able to protect me, how could I do it?

But in that moment, those fears fade. I realize what I am feeling is maternal longing. It is as if biology has touched me with her magic wand, and my ovaries have awoken. The change in my body and mind from not wanting to be a mother to wanting a child is sudden and absolute.

Within sixteen months, at thirty-one, I will welcome my daughter earthside.

I will have become the thing that scared me the most: a mother.

* * *

When I started down the path of my so-called "cancer journey," I was surrounded by societal enthusiasm and a virtual pep rally of pink confetti and messaging. "Kick cancer's ass!" "Cancer messed with the wrong woman!" "You're the strongest person I know!" "You've got this!"

Four months into chemo, I'm not so sure I belong at this pep rally anymore. Someone's ass is getting kicked but I'm not so sure it's cancer's. I finally look like what they said I was all along: a cancer patient. Seeing myself in the mirror, I study the raccoon-eyed, hairless, moon-faced baby looking back. Everything but the breast housing the cancer hurts: my head, my stomach, my hands. The shots I get to boost my white blood cell count ahead of infusions make my bones ache. Even my finger and toenails haven't escaped the wreckage; every day another one turns black and falls off. I'm not throwing up, but the nausea is so insidious that I hang my head over the toilet, wishing for even one moment of relief.

My chemo infusions happen every third Tuesday for five and a half months.

The first few days after an infusion, I feel pretty good thanks to a potent cocktail of steroids and premeds. However, the Benadryl knocks me out during the infusion itself despite my best efforts to stay awake. I'm a remote conference producer for a firm in New York. My manager has been extremely supportive, telling me to work only as I'm able, but I can't allow cancer to steal my ability to meet a deadline, at least not yet. So I work through the fog.

Later, I'll look back and laugh that, of course, the youngest person in the chemo lounge is the one who can't see cancer as an invitation to pause. Each infusion day, I pack fingerless mittens, extra socks, hot bone broth, and my heavy laptop into my bag. As the nurse tucks me under warm blankets, I settle in to research a conference agenda for Medicare insurance executives. It isn't long before I'm asleep like the rest of the cancer patients in our La-Z-Boy recliners.

Eight hours later, I'm on my way home, and the steroids are kicking in. People in the cancer community joke that infusion night, when you're home bouncing off the walls from the steroids, is when you clean your whole house. I don't clean—I write. I sit on the edge of my bed, wide-eyed at 2 a.m., watching the wind whip through the oak tree in the backyard, mirroring my tumultuous thoughts. Beside me sleep Joe and Nia while my brain clangs, full of adrenaline, full of what-ifs, full of grief. My fingers fly over my keyboard, barely able to keep up with my thoughts. I am desperate to get them all out of my head, to set the anxiety down at least for a little bit. Those late-night sessions turn into raw, soul-baring blog posts I share with family and friends.

By day four, the side effects have arrived in full force. For the next week, I'm exhausted and fighting to feel human. My world is reduced to trudging from bed to bathroom to giant beanbag in the living room. Never a napper before, now I watch the clock to see if it's acceptable to go back to bed yet.

A week later, I start to feel better, and each day I climb further out of the pit and fog of side effects. When I finally stand on the surface again, the next infusion day arrives. As the infusions tick by, it's getting harder and harder to force myself into the chemo lounge. My body and brain rebel against the accumulated poison.

Studying my body in the mirror, I touch my breast, cupping the lump in my hand. Is it shrinking? Is the chemo working?

I'm forced to take a big step back in the amount of hands-on time I spend with my daughter during this time. Before cancer, I spent a couple of solo hours with Nia each morning while Joe slept in. Once he was up, she'd transition to him, and I would work for several hours down the hall in the spare bedroom-slash-home office. Then she was back to me, and Joe went off to work the late shift at the library.

Now I reluctantly surrender: I cannot do hours of physically and emotionally demanding parenting. My overflowing calendar of doctor appointments and chemo infusions means long days away from Nia, followed by weeks of recovery that force me into bed. I'm heartbroken, and Nia is angry—not just at me but the whole world. My once easy-going child throws tantrums at bedtime, refuses naps, and has become picky about food. Friends with older children console me by saying she is simply trying to control what little she can. She cries so much each day at preschool that she now regularly sits in the director's office until I can fetch her. It hurts to know how angry she is, but I understand. I am angry too. Before cancer, I was the mom who made breakfast-for-dinner picnics in the living room, the mom who taught Nia how to identify trees in the forest, the mom who never said no to just one more book. Now, I'm a mom who naps.

Visions of Ingrid taking to her bed fill my head. Birthdays and Christmases would be suddenly declared over at the slightest misstep. She would throw up her hands, or throw down the Christmas tree, or throw a full plate of dinner off the deck, then stomp to her bed, pulling the covers over her head. Martin, Dale, Kyle, and I were then supposed to quietly enter her bedroom, apologize, and beg her to return to us. She would only emerge when she was ready. Sometimes, within hours; sometimes, weeks would go by. Whether she was out of bed and terrorizing me, or in bed casting a heavy gloom over the house, I walked on eggshells.

"Be awake when I get home, Mama," Nia always says before reluctantly leaving for preschool or a playdate.

I want to comply. I don't want to be a mom who takes to her bed, forcing the whole family to tiptoe around a darkened bedroom. I don't want the bedroom to become the beating heart of our fear, like it was in my childhood.

The comparison is inescapable. I'm in bed, just like Ingrid was. But the difference, I realize, is this: Ingrid retreated in anger. I retreat in pain. Ingrid weaponized her illness by making it a punishment for the rest of us. I am trying, however imperfectly, to shield Nia from mine. I'm not hiding from her. I'm fighting to return. Still, the fear that I'm repeating Ingrid's patterns haunts me. That fear was part of what kept me from becoming a mother in the first place.

* * *

During my treatment time, Nia spends a lot of time with her grandparents. Phil and Pam live in a second-floor apartment above our house. Years ago, before our wedding, Joe, his parents, and I intentionally decided to live in a multi-generational home. We imagined helping them as they aged. We didn't know I would be the one needing help so soon into our living arrangement. Now, Nia spends a lot of time upstairs with her "Bama and Baba." Sometimes we've planned for them to watch her, but other times, she runs upstairs on a whim for an hour to be read to, snuggled, or for a special Bama snack. When she's satiated, she runs back down to me.

These days, as the weight of chemo accumulates, I'm stretched thin, even with preschool and grandparents nearby. I'm not always able to "Be awake, Mama!" So I piece together a calendar of playdates for Nia, a kind of cousin to the Meal Train that keeps our porch stocked with love in colorful Tupperware squares. It feels strange to ask people to take my child. I so desperately want to be her primary person—to be the mom Ingrid couldn't be for me. What I fear most is not the illness itself, but what it might steal: my presence, attentiveness, and ability to hold Nia close in the ways that matter. I'm terrified the mother-daughter bond is so fragile that even a mild breeze—much less cancer—could crack its surface. And in our case, that crack might grow and grow until all that's left is distance, leaving us emotionally estranged, the way I was from my own mother.

If I have to ask for help raising my child, I will do it with intention, I decide. Deliberately. Lovingly. On my terms. I've learned that when we decide to act with purpose, the universe often shows up and gives us exactly what we need. For me, it showed up in the form of an NPR interview.

The segment was with *New York Times* bestselling author and television host Bruce Feiler. As a young dad, Bruce explained, he received a shattering cancer diagnosis. In the aftermath, he found himself consumed by a singular, haunting question: Who would be there for his wife and daughters if he were gone? So he reached out to six men who helped shape him and asked them to be present in the lives of his daughters during his cancer treatment, with the idea that they would continue to be there if he passed away. Ultimately, his cancer went into remission, and he wrote a book called *The Council of Dads: A Story of Family, Friendship & Learning How to Live.*

I realized that while I ached for all the things my mom couldn't give me, I was raised by many other strong, generous women who each gave me parts of themselves. There was my beloved, white-haired, fairy-like kindergarten teacher Betty Peck; my chic, independent aunt Berit; my crystal and sage-loving neighbor Joan, a Manhattan transplant with her black curls and bright red lipstick. Later, my mother-in-law Pam became a mom to me, teaching me by example and gently guiding me toward being the mom and wife I am today. I am so lucky to have had these women in my life.

After listening to the interview, I started to think about forming my own "council of mothers" for Nia. At first, the idea was a "just in case"—if I didn't survive, I wanted Nia to have more than memories. But soon, it became something else: a way to care for her right now, during my cancer fighting, in the space between good days and bed days. Maybe instead of believing I need to be Nia's everything and grieving that I can't do it all during cancer, maybe this is an opportunity to welcome in other strong women to help mold and guide her.

I decide my council must be people that Nia is comfortable with already. They must be people who share similar parenting and discipline beliefs as me, and if we are on different pages when it comes to discipline, they have to be people whom I know won't do anything with Nia I would disapprove of. This idea of safety is paramount given my abuse background and the deep-rooted fears that kept me from having a child for so long: that I wouldn't always be able to protect her. Nia's council of mothers has to be made up of people who can offer a safe environment for play, exploration, big emotions, and deep conversation. My girl is working through a lot, and I need her to be with women who can respect that and nurture her. I look to my extended family, the parents of Nia's friends, and my female friends who have known me the longest. To my surprise, the friends who knew me before I became a mother are the ones to whom I'm most drawn. This is where I begin to build the council.

There's Megan, who lives in San Francisco; no kids yet. She likes to say her name rhymes with *vegan*. My oldest friend, Megan knows where the bodies are buried. She's been by my side since we were five. She witnessed my childhood, including abuse first-hand, let me follow her to college, didn't judge me when I transferred to another university a semester later, was my wedding planner, and sat in the front pew with me at Ingrid's funeral.

Michelle is next. We have been friends since seventh-grade band. She was the first chair flute while I was dead-last chair flute, which meant I sat right behind her. She never once made me feel ashamed to be last. Instead, it was the perfect arrangement to laugh and joke together all band period long. Later, when Ingrid pulled me out of school to homeschool, Michelle didn't forget me. Years later, without the benefit of the Internet, she somehow tracked me down. Ultimately, we became housemates and colleagues, our days bookended by 4 a.m. trips to the gym and late-night ice cream binges in bed together.

Lastly, there is Erin. Erin lives in a converted barn in a beautiful slough. Occasionally, owls stand on the skylight high above her bed. We've been friends since college. Erin is a marine biologist-turned-middle-school teacher who drives a purring, yellow diesel Volkswagen Karmann Ghia with a surfboard on top and Tom Petty leaking out the open windows. No children herself yet, Erin grew up with a single mom and has taught me a great deal about what it means to be strong and independent.

These three women have lifted me up, dried my tears, and made me laugh like no one else can, time and time again. We've talked about absolutely everything and experienced a great deal of life together too. And now, as I face my most significant life challenge, here they are again. Lifting me up. Drying my tears. Making me laugh. This time it isn't just me though. Now there is Nia, and they are doing the same for her. Distracting her. Making her laugh. Listening when she needs to share. Playing tag and chase when she just needs to burn off some energy, and cooking with her. They are not replacements for me. They are reinforcements.

I'd like to think that had I not become sick, I'd have encouraged my pre-Nia friends to spend time with her one-on-one, but I'm not sure if I would have. Being sick has made this a necessity. They step in when I have to step out, providing her with all that a truly good mother does: love, compassion, understanding, joy, redirection.

They are me when I can't be, but they are also themselves with Nia and that's a tremendous gift. Building this council of mothers has shown me that there can be strength in the breaking. Cancer broke our family open, and what poured in was love.

* * *

It's been five days since my mastectomy to remove my left breast. Five days since Whitney came from Montana to care for Nia. Five days of Whitney asking Nia if she wants to see me and five days of a short, defiant "No" in response.

Five days of profound grief for both of us.

And then, slowly, she comes back to me. As suddenly as she pulled away, she returns. One night, she decides to sleep with Joe and me, simple as that.

We dim the lights, turn on the white noise machine and night light. We settle into our California King bed together, and Joe picks up the bedtime book they started before my surgery. Nia lies between us. As Joe reads, I close my eyes and feel something I had not dared hope for: my daughter begins to inch toward me, literally closing the chasm with her small body.

First, her head leans against mine, her hair brushing my short, barely-there lashes. Then, her hand strokes my cheek before traveling up to rub the new, spiky hair sprouting from my scalp.

Next, her hand begins to explore my wounded chest. First, on the surface of my T-shirt, then after several minutes, her hand slowly creeps inside my shirt, and her fingers gently explore my bandages. She traces along the smooth tape and the soft, white gauze. Lightly, she feels along the thin plastic tubing of the drains. She touches my stomach and feels the places on my chest that are not sealed in bandages.

And then she exhales.

Her whole body relaxes as she nestles her forehead into my neck. Joe reads on. I don't move. I let the tears slide silently from the corners of my eyes toward my ears. I hold my breath, afraid that any shift might startle this small, brave animal back into her shell.

I had believed the mother-daughter bond was always one bad moment away from breaking. But now I see it differently: when it's built with presence and care, it can bend, stretch—even through cancer—and not break.

What I didn't understand then was that giving Nia space to grieve, without demanding she worship at the feet of my suffering, was the proof that I had already begun to break the cycle I was so scared of. I will never know what our relationship might have been had I not had cancer. In the years since my diagnosis, more grief has come: my father-in-law Phil's death; Joe's sister's early-onset dementia unfolding inside our home; Martin's death. In the seven years between Ingrid's death and his own, Martin also went to work breaking our family cycles. Through healing his painful past with Ingrid, including accompanying me to several therapy appointments, he grew into a wonderful grandfather. He became the loving, nurturing, and healthy dad I longed for. Like me, I think he always had an idea of the parent he wanted to be, and finally, that version emerged from the rubble of his relationship. I'm so glad it wasn't too late for us to build something new. I asked him once how he felt about me calling him by his first name. He said he liked it and that it represented a new chapter for us in his mind too. We made a lifetime of memories in those seven years before he passed away.

I know now that none of us parent in perfect conditions. There will always be outside forces battering the fortress of the family and our notions of who we desire to be as parents. I know now: we don't stay strong because we manage to keep those forces out. We stay strong by letting ourselves bend and adjust; we let the world in, and let it shape us.

I've learned there will always be echoes of the ones who made us, no matter how hard we work to break generational cycles. While I have been vigilant in keeping Ingrid's voice out of my mouth, she still lingers in my mind. However, cancer didn't turn me into her against my will. Quite the opposite. It showed me that Ingrid had a choice and she did not choose me. I have also learned that fighting cancer does not have to disrupt my healing from my past. In a lot of ways, I found myself in the fire of cancer. I was terrified that the healthy motherhood I created for myself and Nia would slip through my fingers—that cancer would tear apart the true bond I'd longed my whole life to build. Instead, cancer tightened my grip on my convictions, and against everything I feared, Nia came back to me. Not because I forced her out of a fear of abandonment like Ingrid felt every day of her life, but instead because I learned there is safety in taking space to heal. I didn't leave or vanish into my illness, I didn't hold my daughter hostage to my suffering, and I didn't punish her for her grief.

Over Nia's head, as she rests against me, I slowly turn toward Joe. He looks up from the book and meets my gaze. He smiles.

With two days to spare before Whitney leaves, my daughter has come back to me. I haven't been replaced, and I haven't failed. Cancer is not the end of us. Instead, this is the beautiful breaking open to a deeper bond.

We are so not fucked. We are forged.

AUTHOR BIO

April Stearns is the founder and editor in chief of *Wildfire Journal &*
Writing Community.

A lifelong writer who landed her first memoir-based magazine
cover story at just sixteen, April worked for her college newspaper
(*City on the Hill* at the University of California at Santa Cruz) and
then went on to work for her local newspaper (*The Sentinel*, Santa
Cruz, CA) following graduation. Before long, she was lured to other
writing jobs "over the hill" from Santa Cruz in Silicon Valley during
the tech boom of the early 2000s.

However, in 2012, in the midst of this career, April was diagnosed
with Stage 3 breast cancer at age thirty-five. Four years later, while
struggling to "go back to normal" and find others in similar circumstances, April launched *Wildfire Journal & Writing Community* as a
way for younger people to tell and read breast cancer stories.

Since 2016, April has guided hundreds of writers through the
Wildfire expressive writing and memoir writing workshops and published more than fifty issues of *Wildfire Journal*.

April believes strongly that helping others tell their stories has
the dramatic effect of turning a traumatic cancer experience into an
empowering one. April lives with her husband and young daughter in
Santa Cruz. Although she loves town life, she also likes to get away
from all the hustle and bustle whenever she can to hike in the woods,
but writing memoir remains April's purest escape.

MELISSA ANDERSEN

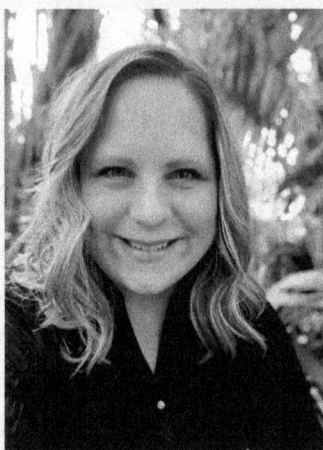

As a first-generation college student with everything to lose, I couldn't afford the vulnerability needed to process grief. Success meant escape toward a life I dreamed of. I presented myself as strong and capable, distancing myself from the small-town stereotypes I feared others saw in me. Showing too much grief felt like a sign of weakness, a lack of grit. This shell, however, would eventually crack as I confronted my mortality. In what felt like an unraveling, I would eventually begin to see that anger and grief weren't signs of weakness. They were proof I was still alive.

BECOMING THE SOIL THE SEEDS NEED

A Journey Through Cancer, Prairie Fires, and Learning What It Means to Be Fully Human

My muscles tense as I scan the room, topless. My reconstructed breasts are exposed for the whole world to see, each one marked by scars that resemble crosshairs. I think about the irony that I have been caught in my own life and death line of fire as a result of a terrible disease. *Is this really happening?* I wonder, not for the first time, as I look around the tattoo shop in Olympia, Washington. My partner Daren and I traveled from Minnesota, and while we've come the farthest to be here, this is only one small, yet symbolic, part of the journey we've been on together. I am one out of five breast cancer survivors, all chosen to receive a mastectomy tattoo through Personal Ink (P.ink), a program aimed at empowering women as we reclaim our bodies after breast cancer. The whole thing seems like a dream, and I look around the space, at the images the other women designed with their assigned artists, and then at Daren, who knows me better than anyone, as he studies the stenciled outline being transferred to my chest. "It's so you," he assures me with his trademark smile.

So much intention and care from volunteers went into planning this day, and I find myself wanting to savor each moment. While the tattoo shop includes the usual decor of seemingly random and dark artifacts, including a real coffin displayed like a collector's item, the energy is anything but dark. I find amusement in the idea of a coffin watching as five women who have stared death in the eyes celebrate their survival. Fresh flowers and balloons in various shades of pink adorn a table filled with food—charcuterie, salmon, fruit, and pastries—spread out to keep us nourished for the day, donated by local businesses. I'm too excited to eat at first, but I take inventory in my head of the things that I plan to come back for, because anyone who knows me would agree that I never pass up charcuterie or pastries. A playlist of uplifting music, including Rachel Platten's "Fight Song," helps set the mood as we get comfortable for the afternoon of taking back our bodies and metamorphosis ahead.

I tune into the buzz of the tattoo gun as I steady my breath and try to stay still. A young woman named Natalee has offered her time and talent for free to help me transform my scarred chest into a beautiful swallowtail butterfly flitting around zinnia flowers, just like the ones I know from my summer garden. Her design captures my ideas perfectly, and after a short conversation with her, I know she was meant to be my artist.

As Natalee begins her work and the first ink is injected, a cascade of emotions washes over me. A chill creeps through my body as I recall the last time I lay awake on a table, waiting for a needle to pierce the skin of my chest. While it has been over four years, all the difficulties that have brought me to this point in my journey come flooding back.

For the first time in a long time, I can honestly say to myself, *I'm grateful to be alive for this.* Teary-eyed, I smile at Natalee and nod my head to let her know I am more than ready.

* * *

I lay in the darkened ultrasound room, trying to focus on the image of an English-style garden in full bloom on the suspended ceiling tiles above me. I had been in this room two days earlier when I was in for the investigation of a painful lump I had found in my right breast a month prior. The radiologist had just gone over what to expect during the procedure. I would feel a needle being inserted, and then several quick, sharp stabs as they took a few core-needle biopsies of my lump.

Gripping my hands into tight fists, I tried to imagine walking through the garden pictured on the ceiling as the needle punctured my breast. A sharp sting surged through my body, and I was immediately ripped away from my imagined walk in the garden and back to my scary reality. Unable to choke back the tears, I surrendered, allowing the floodgates to open. As I wept in fear, the radiologist matter-of-factly reminded me to breathe and stay as still as I could. It was as if she had no idea what this moment meant for me. Up until then, I hadn't let myself believe it might be cancer. The biopsy, however, made it all seem very real. My heart raced, as my body trembled. *Is this really happening? Breast cancer? I just turned forty-one. That's too young, right? And this virus—this pandemic. Fuck.*

I felt the nurse's hand gently on my shoulder—a steady, quiet anchor. "You're doing great," she said, her voice a soft counterpoint to the radiologist's more clinical focus as she worked methodically, taking several samples from the underside of my right breast. When the needle was finally removed, the nurse told me to take my time. Once they left the room, I sat at the edge of the exam table, breathing deeply to gather myself. I did my best to clean up the streaks of mascara left from my tears. Too sore to wear it, I stuffed my bra into my purse. Back in the safety of my car in the dimly lit parking garage, tears came again. It was March 18, 2020—the beginning of the COVID pandemic. I wept the whole way home, fearing what was to come.

*   *   *

I went back and forth between my laptop and my phone. Distracted and anxious, I couldn't focus on work. It was the fourth day of working from home because of the COVID lockdown. There hadn't been time to set up a home office for me yet, so my things were sprawled out at the dining room table—stacks of picture books covered in Post-it notes for a curriculum project, a notebook, a set of colorful pens, and my essential beverages—coffee and water.

I stared out the window as a steady rain gently washed away winter's grime. It had been raining all day, and it smelled like spring. Scientists call this earthy and pleasant scent petrichor, produced when certain bacteria are released from the soil as it rains after a dry period, an aroma I'd always loved. I couldn't help but wonder if it would now carry with it the memory of that moment. My mind drifted into a daydream, trying to predict how I would handle whatever the results of yesterday's biopsy would be. As morning turned to midday and then to afternoon, I grew more anxious about getting the call I was expecting to receive. I checked my phone repeatedly to see if I'd missed it somehow.

When my phone finally rang just after 3:00 p.m., I took a deep breath and stood up from my chair. Gathering all my courage, I answered the call, surprised that it was my primary care doctor rather than the radiology department. After asking how I was doing, she informed me that my lump was a malignant tumor, just over three centimeters. I paced rapidly between the dining and living rooms, my dog Barley right on my heels, following me back and forth. For a moment, I couldn't remember if malignant meant cancerous or not. *She hadn't said cancer, had she?* She went on. The diagnosis was stage 2, invasive ductal carcinoma that was HER2-positive and aggressive. She described what HER2-positive means—that cancer cells in my breast were making too many HER2 proteins, amplifying their division and causing an aggressively growing tumor. The bottom line was simple: I had breast cancer.

I stopped pacing and stood there, frozen in time. Everything around me disappeared for a moment, and I felt my heart pound, heavy in my chest. Realizing that I had been holding my breath, I tried to breathe, but the air felt too thick to draw in.

The doctor assured me that it was unlikely to have spread beyond my breast. She calmly explained that at my age, I could beat this with the good treatments available. I remained quiet, and to fill the silence, she mentioned lifestyle changes that would increase the effectiveness of treatment, such as changing my diet and exercising more. What I should eat for breakfast or the number of steps I should take every day felt like trivial details. I stopped listening. I don't remember the rest of the call.

After a moment of dissociation where I pictured my funeral and wondered who would show up, I returned to my body. Still standing in the dining room, I met eyes with Barley, who stood at my feet, staring at me, wide-eyed and panting. They say dogs can sense human emotion, but I believe Barley is what Daren calls a superfeeler, just like me. Unlike me, however, Barley shows all his cards and allows himself to express his emotions without holding back, something I still had yet to learn.

I needed to go downstairs and tell Daren, who was on a call with a coworker. He took one look at my face and told his coworker he'd call them back. I blurted out, "I have cancer," and that was all I could say before the tears took over. He pulled me close and held me. We stood in the basement, embraced in a tight hug as I sobbed, soaking his T-shirt with my salty tears.

That night, I didn't sleep despite being emotionally and physically exhausted. I had spent the rest of the day calling loved ones to break the news, crying often. Restless, I lay awake as the hours passed, wondering what I had done to deserve cancer. My mind spun with questions so fast I felt nauseous, like a carnival ride I wish I could stop. *Will I get to see my family again before I get too sick? What if I get COVID? Is this the beginning of how it ends for me? Will I survive this? Why is this happening to me? Is it my fault? What did I do to deserve this?*

* * *

Daren drove down the tree-lined streets of our neighborhood while I sat quietly next to him in the passenger seat. Barley, who had taken his post in the backseat, was looking out the window, the fluffy golden hair on top of his head bouncing as we moved onto the highway. It was my first day of chemotherapy. I hadn't slept the night before, jittery from the steroids I'd taken to help curb the inevitable side effects. I didn't know how I'd feel after the long day ahead, so Daren offered to drive me and pick me up. I was to be there just before 9:00 a.m. and expected to be there most of the day. That was all I knew.

I had packed a green canvas tote with things that would make me more comfortable for the day: a handmade blanket from friends, crackers and peanut butter, a banana, water, a book, and my journal. I held onto the love and encouragement I'd received leading up to this day as my lifeline. The day before, my coworkers had even shown up outside my house, their cars decorated with signs they had made to cheer me on, filling my neighborhood with music by the Indigo Girls, my favorite band.

Reminding myself that I could do hard things, I shut the door on unpleasant emotions, a skill I'd mastered long ago. This coping mechanism had served me well in the past, or so I thought, so naturally, I clung to it during this traumatic time. I just wanted to get through the day.

Before I was ready, we pulled up in front of the door of the hospital. With tears in my eyes, I gave Daren a kiss and Barley a pat on the head. I didn't want to go in, and I wished more than anything that Daren could come with me. I'd known people who had chemotherapy before, and they always had a family member or close friend with them for support, but because of the restrictions surrounding COVID, I was not allowed a companion. While a steady stream of text messages came in from friends and family wishing me strength for the day ahead, I hated that I had to face the day alone.

After checking in and getting my blood drawn, I saw my oncologist briefly before being escorted to the infusion room, a semi-circle of reclining chairs facing large windows that overlooked bird feeders in the foreground of a wooded area. I looked around to see who I was going to be spending my day with. Among the half-a-dozen-or-so other patients, I could only guess, but it looked like I was the youngest one of the day.

I received infusions of four different drugs—two chemotherapy drugs to kill the cancer and two to help target the overexpression of the HER2 receptor protein that was feeding it. I found the whole thing quite surreal. Nurses dressed in what looked like hazmat suits hooked up bags of poison to my line, and one toxic liquid after another was pumped into my body through a port installed near my heart the week before. "You're not getting any wimpy chemo, my dear!" one nurse commented through her face mask.

Nurses monitored me closely since it was my first dose, so I was the last chemo patient of the day to finish. I texted Daren that it was time to come and get me, and continued watching out the window, hoping the wild turkeys I saw foraging for food earlier would return so I could get a picture on my phone. I thought about all the things I would tell Daren on our way home: about how I had been ordered to flush the toilet twice after using it to minimize the exposure of toxins to others and about the hazmat suits.

After dark, we took a drive to a nearby open field to see the pink supermoon. Sitting in silence in the car, we stared at the large moon for a while, trying to distract ourselves from our current reality. The full moon appeared more orange than pink, glowing as if it were on fire. I stared in awe, sensing a strange kinship, as if the fire in the moon mirrored the one burning in my body, a vibration deep in my core. I was wide awake, aware of every sensation, my blood humming through my veins with electricity—something I'd never felt before. *Maybe it's the pull of the full moon,* I thought. *More likely, the steroids.* I wondered how long the fire inside me would stay. I didn't know what it meant, but it felt significant. With one chemo down and five to go, it was only the beginning, and fire and I were about to become well acquainted.

Like unwanted guests that I had begrudgingly allowed in, the side effects began to make a mess of my body several days posttreatment, and I learned firsthand that chemo was my hell. Nausea, diarrhea, mouth and foot sensitivity, bone pain, and a rash that spread from my chest to my face became new sensations to manage in my new reality.

My sense of smell changed, and I could no longer sleep next to Daren, for something about his body chemistry made me nauseous during that time. I lost nearly fifteen pounds in the three weeks between my first two chemo cycles. At any other time, I would've welcomed the weight loss, but my oncologist chided me that chemo is not a weight loss plan.

After my first chemo treatment, my scalp became increasingly more tingly and sensitive each day. Nearly two weeks after the first dose, I stood in the shower, letting the warm water run over my face. In anticipation that I'd be losing my hair, Daren had taken off the underside of my short bob with a set of clippers borrowed from a friend. The plan had been to buzz it all, so there would be less of my hair falling out on my pillow or clothes, but I just couldn't go through with it. All of the changes to my body seemed to be happening so fast, and holding onto my hair as long as I could seemed like a way to maintain a sense of normalcy.

That morning, as I wet my hair under the spray of warm water, clumps of it came out in handfuls. I burst into tears as I watched piles of hair make their way down the drain. I stood, sobbing, as the water carried my hair away. I knew this moment was coming, yet somehow I was still caught off guard. I tried to tell myself that it was just hair, that it would grow back, but the loss felt deeper than that.

I washed the rest of my body as I continued to cry. Even my pubic hair came out on my washcloth. I hadn't realized that losing my hair meant I would lose all the hair on my body. No one had told me that would happen, and I felt embarrassed that I had been so naive. Eventually, I'd even lose my eyebrows and most of my eyelashes.

I turned off the water and opened the shower curtain. Still teary, I grabbed my towel and caught my reflection in the mirror. I stood there staring at myself, dripping wet, unable to look away. My hair, now in thin patches, barely covered my head; I realized the outside of me matched how bad the chemo was making me feel on the inside. I now looked sick, instead of just feeling sick. Weepy and raw, I finished getting ready for work and tried to push the heavy feelings aside.

As my body continued to change, a deep sense of grief that I had tried to ignore found its way in through the cracks of everything I was trying to hold together. It had been a year since I left my position as a middle school teacher to join an education nonprofit led by a dear friend. Perhaps it was triggered by a sense of all that I felt I lost control over in a short period, or the fact that I was at the first anniversary of the decision to leave the classroom, that hit me. Either way, I found myself deeply missing my former students, my former coworkers, and the school community that had been my home for ten years—all pieces of my former life, before cancer.

I questioned whether I'd made the right decision to leave, even though the burnout had been real, and I looked forward to a fresh start doing work I was passionate about. While I loved my students and my school, I had struggled with boundaries, allowing my work to consume me. I had stopped sleeping well, spending countless nights lying awake, worrying about things I had no control over. Those nights awake rendered me exhausted all the time, and some mornings, I fought back tears as I drove to school. *Had I not made a change, the pandemic and my cancer would likely have forced me out anyway, so at least I got to do it on my terms,* I kept reminding myself. Even so, I carried shame for not being strong enough to handle being a teacher. I felt silly for grieving this loss a year later, especially when I had so much more to worry about, not realizing the compounded loss I was experiencing.

The next month, following my third of six intense chemo treatments, George Floyd, an unarmed Black man, was murdered by a Minneapolis police officer just miles from my home. In the following days, protests erupted nearby. The constant pulsing of helicopters and intermittent pops of flashbangs in the distance made it harder for me to focus on rest and taking care of myself in my sickest posttreatment days. My heart sank when I learned that one of the officers involved was a former student of mine. I remembered him as a middle schooler, navigating adolescence and identity. *How had we failed him?* I felt a sense of culpability, wishing I had done more for my former students. As I watched a long overdue racial reckoning unfold on TV and social media, and my friends attended protests and marches, I felt like I wasn't doing enough while physically unable to do more in the moment.

Facing cancer amidst the isolation of a global pandemic was already more than I believed I could hold. Layer on the surfacing grief of losing my identity as a teacher, a role that had shaped so much of who I was, along with the distress over George Floyd's murder, and I was overwhelmed by a flood of sorrow, anger, and uncertainty. I was mourning the person I used to be in a world that no longer felt familiar. I was drowning, being pulled down by the heavy undercurrent of my insecurities.

I often found myself angry, mostly at my body. It wasn't fair, yet I didn't fully admit how betrayed I felt by it. I stuffed the disappointment down like a polite dinner guest would lie about hating the food. I declared how badly I was going to kick cancer's ass, even when all I wanted to do was cry, scream, and have others sit with me to acknowledge my pain. Aware that everyone else was grappling with the crisis of the pandemic, I tried to remain upbeat when friends would check on me and tried not to ask for too much help.

For most of my life, I worked hard to control difficult emotions. I swallowed anger, buried grief, and called it strength. Anger, especially, felt forbidden—something dangerous. As a child, I watched it twist adults into versions of themselves I never wanted to become: volatile, alcoholic, or victims of deeply held shame. As a first-generation college student with everything to lose, I couldn't afford the vulnerability needed to process grief. Success meant escape toward a life I dreamed of. I presented myself as strong and capable, distancing myself from the small-town stereotypes I feared others saw in me. Showing too much grief felt like a sign of weakness, a lack of grit. This shell, however, would eventually crack as I confronted my mortality. In what felt like an unraveling, I would eventually begin to see that anger and grief weren't signs of weakness. They were proof I was still alive.

It's funny how the universe has a way of making sure we learn the lessons we need to, and how our bodies have so much to teach us if we allow ourselves to listen. The emotions I had internalized as negative, such as anger or grief, would be the ones I'd be forced to accept as part of being human, and if there is anything I have learned from this journey, it is what it means to be fully human.

* * *

Daren and I sat on a blanket under the shade of old oak trees in a city park, listening to children play and groups of friends laugh around us. We had done a lot of things in our eighteen years of marriage, but never anything like the last four months, and our anniversary dinner had never been on a picnic blanket. I tried to eat the fish sandwich and French fries—takeout Daren had gotten us from the seafood restaurant located in the park. Since chemo, most foods felt like shag carpet in my mouth, and this was no different.

As we shared our anniversary picnic under the trees, their leaves dancing gently above us, I was reminded of how much my partner loved me. He didn't care that I was bald or pale, while my cheeks always seemed to be puffy and flushed, with bags weighing down my eyes. He saw not only my physical decline, but also my strength, even when I couldn't. I realized how lucky I was to have known this kind of love. Cancer had begun to transform our relationship in ways we weren't prepared for, and he became my caregiver, my rock. We faced chaos and uncertainty together, and we grew closer than ever.

As Daren and I sat there together, I was intentional in taking in all that I could that was joyful about that moment, and I became struck by the coexistence of joy and pain. Life was about learning how to live in this juxtaposition, and I was just beginning to find awe in its complexity.

There were plenty of low days, where fatigue and brain fog took the wheel, and I lived too close to the toilet and too far from what I wanted for myself. Some days, I struggled to find the motivation to get out of bed, and tears came easily. At the same time, there were also bright spots that kept me going. My zinnia gardens burst with blooms, drawing in more butterflies than ever before, including my favorites— the yellow swallowtails—as if they knew I needed them that summer. Love arrived from all directions: friends, family, old students, even strangers. My brother called each week just to catch up and listen, and our bond, once strained, quietly mended. I called my mom during the day, knowing she'd answer. Though the pandemic kept us apart, our family text thread became a lifeline—full of jokes, silly pictures, whatever it took to make each other laugh. Somehow, humor became its own kind of medicine.

* * *

The evening before my surgery, bilateral mastectomies, I stood alone, topless in my bedroom, staring at my breasts in the full-length mirror. I thought about messages I'd received as a child about the sexualization of women's bodies and the importance of modesty, such as how a girl should always sit with her legs together or how men would think that showing cleavage was sexy. I never understood those things, but maybe it's where some of my distrust of my own body began. In that moment, though, I quieted those thoughts. I was just about to lose part of my body, and I felt entitled to this time with it. I grinned in defiance and took out my phone.

I took dozens of selfies of my breasts as I said goodbye to them, embracing the moment as sacred and necessary. The whole time leading up to that point, I hadn't considered how much the loss of this part of my body would shake me. After all, even though I was a late bloomer, my dense breasts were often a royal pain in the ass. Supportive bras to lift my double-Ds were expensive, and I struggled to find swimsuits that held them in place. As each menstrual cycle approached, my breasts swelled with a deep, aching pain, and taking off my bra brought me close to tears. I didn't have children, so I wasn't using them for what they were intended for, and I hated that our society had sexualized women's breasts so much. Along with choosing the option that would give me the lowest chances of recurrence, I had convinced myself that having mastectomies would be a relief.

Although the decision to let go of my breasts was surprisingly easy, the choice to reconstruct pulled me into weeks of restless circling, like a bird unsure where to land. Plastic surgery felt unnatural, like chasing something I had already surrendered. I wanted to be one of those women who moved boldly through life flat-chested, unbothered by stares or silence. When I asked friends what they thought, responses ranged from, "It's a chance for a nice boob job," to "Are you sure you're ready to go flat?" Daren, steady as ever, only cared that I felt whole. He'd love me either way. When I took the time to look inward in stillness, searching for clarity, I was able to admit that I felt more at home in a body with breasts and opted for implants—not to cling to some past version of me, and not for anyone else, but because I'd truly miss my breasts.

* * *

One morning, about a month after surgery, I was sitting at the kitchen table having breakfast alone, while Daren worked in the next room. The season was shifting, and the cold morning left a layer of frost to remind us that winter was on its way. Like my mood, the late-October sky was gray and heavy.

As I sipped my hot coffee, I stared out the window at the back-yard gardens. A feeling of sadness surfaced. While I had always loved the fact that living in Minnesota meant experiencing all four distinct seasons, I dreaded the return of winter that year. I felt cheated out of my summer, for I had spent most of it navigating appointments or reeling from treatment and unable to enjoy the longer days. The pandemic lingered on, and after seven months, we remained cautious and isolated, terrified that COVID would be the thing to kill me. Now, as the weather grew colder, gathering with friends outdoors would be more difficult. I worried the holiday season would come and we wouldn't get the chance to be with family after the year we could use it the most.

The afternoon before, Daren and I had cut down all the zinnias from our garden in the backyard to save as many as possible from the predicted frost. Setting aside half the flower heads for drying to ensure seeds for next year's crop, multiple mason jars and vases of zinnias were scattered throughout the house, their cheery colors of pinks, reds, oranges, and yellows working hard to brighten every single room.

I studied the green vase of zinnias in front of me on the table, trying to imagine what the flowers would be thinking about as they overlooked their former home in the garden just beyond the kitchen window, now just an empty plot of soil under scattered leaves. *Were they relieved to have been rescued from the frost? Or were they dreading their inevitable fate of slowly wilting as they faced death?* I noticed one half-open bud, peeking out hesitantly among the others, as if unsure whether it was even worth blooming in a vase where no butterfly would ever come to complete the cycle, to give the bloom her intended purpose.

In a way, the zinnias provided me with a metaphor for how I was feeling. My prognosis was good, I had no evidence of disease. Though I had been rescued from death, there was an ache inside me I hadn't fully faced, and I kept it buried beneath the rush to heal. The pandemic's isolation was wearing on me, and I longed for human connection—for comforting arms to embrace and remind me why it was worth working so hard to stay alive. Treatment and surgery had taken a toll on my body, and I worried about what the future would bring—what my purpose truly was. Over the next few years, however, I would come to realize that a cancer journey doesn't end when the disease is out of your body; there's so much more beyond the treatments.

* * *

"Do you know what today is?" I asked Daren as we sat at the kitchen table, having dinner. He looked at me like he was about to respond with his familiar and clever sense of humor, but after sensing my seriousness, decided not to. "One year ago today was my first day of chemo," I said. I'd been having a lot of one-year-ago-today moments, and Daren finally asked when I'd stop announcing them. I didn't know what to say. *Was it strange to remember them like birthdays or wedding anniversaries?* When I relayed this story to my cancer support group, the facilitator said it made sense because they were all little traumas. That may have been the first time I had heard the word trauma used to describe my breast cancer experience, and somehow naming it as such felt foreign at first. *Was I allowed to use that word—trauma—even with all my privilege?*

I had just finished all my infusions of the drugs to control the expression of HER2 proteins in my cells. It felt so good to be done and on the path to recovery from all those chemicals wreaking havoc on my body. I had received my first COVID vaccine, and in just a couple of days, I'd get my chemo port—the gateway for poison—removed from my chest.

While much good had unfolded, my body was quietly telling a different story. In addition to managing mild lymphedema from having lymph nodes removed, chronic pain crept in and made itself at home in my chest. Scar tissue from capsular contracture had wrapped itself around my implants, hardening where softness should have been. Movement became limited and painful. My uneven reconstructed chest looked awkward in most of my shirts, with my left implant sitting noticeably higher than its partner on the right. I was told it wasn't anything I did wrong, yet I wondered, *Had I made the wrong choice?* I had longed to feel whole again, but instead felt misshapen and unsure. Eventually, I underwent another surgery in an attempt to reclaim comfort and to feel at home in my skin.

As my body continued to betray me, I wondered: *How much grief is allowed when you've survived?* I feared that if I mourned openly, I would seem ungrateful. With the world reopening—graduations, birthdays, retirements—I felt pressure to not only return to the person I was before cancer, but a stronger, more enlightened version of her.

"You look great!" others said, their eyes studying my returning hair, yet much of the time, the acknowledgement seemed to end there.

Just as I longed for space to heal, Daren and I were thrust into caregiving as we tended to aging parents, which brought with it a new set of challenges. There was little room to honor survivorship, let alone the tangled grief that came with it. Instead of compassion, I scolded myself. Grief still felt like a flaw, and disappointment, a kind of selfishness.

A friend and former colleague who had also faced cancer shared a metaphor that stayed with me: "I think dealing with a major health crisis is like going through a mountain range with many hurdles and unexpected challenges. Then, when you come out of the mountain, you realize there is an expanse of prairie extending to the horizon that you have to cross." His words resonated, and they were the validation I needed. I had just emerged from the mountains and was stepping into my prairie. It wouldn't be a steep climb anymore, but the journey ahead would still prove challenging. I tried to remember the beauty prairies hold—tall grasses, wildflowers, bees, and butterflies—so I wouldn't be too discouraged over how far I had left to go. The weight of unspoken grief would slow me, and I knew I'd have to pause, unpack, and let those emotions breathe. I didn't want to miss the magic of the prairie or the lessons waiting in its wide, open space.

I couldn't return to life as it was before cancer, nor did I want to. Somehow, my shell had cracked, and through the cracks, self-compassion began to find its way in. The universe was offering a chance to live more authentically, and I chose to say yes. I committed to healing, even when it felt uncomfortable: months of physical therapy, a regular workout routine, and a wellness program through the iRise Above Foundation, where I discovered the healing properties of creative outlets like art and writing, and most importantly, connection with women who truly understood. I began therapy to face my grief and anger, and slowly leaned into mindfulness, listening to my body with new respect. I started telling myself, *I get to be angry. I get to be disappointed.* I was finally learning to honor my full, human self.

Some weeks, progress came easily. There'd be an easier workout or a stretch of days without tears, and I'd feel proud—like I was finally moving forward. On Fridays, Daren and I held living room dance parties with music blaring and Barley zooming around with his toys. Where we lacked rhythm, we had joy.

Other weeks were heavier. Energy and motivation were just out of reach, and it felt like I was sliding backward. The progress was never linear. But over time, I saw that resilience wasn't about grit—it was about softening and learning to live inside the complexity. The seeds of healing were already there, slowly taking root.

* * *

After cancer treatment, my periods returned with a vengeance—pain sharp enough to cut me down some days. I learned to plan around it, lowering my expectations, again and again. It was even more difficult to explain it to others, and many didn't seem to understand. I didn't either.

Sex became another loss. First my breasts, now my womb—each attempt felt like a tearing apart from the inside out. Pain had taken up residence where pleasure used to live, and although Daren remained endlessly kind and gentle, I grieved the physical intimacy and chemistry we once shared.

For three years, I searched through doctors, tests, and medication, chasing a name for the pain. When the only answer I received was normal perimenopause, a voice inside me persisted, *This is not normal.*

Finally, I found a doctor who suspected endometriosis, a condition in which the same tissue that lines the uterus grows outside of it, binding itself to other organs. With each month's cycle, it would build and bleed, causing pain and violent periods. *Why had no one mentioned this before?* I learned that many women experience a similar path to diagnosis, with the process taking up to ten years or more.

Treatment options were limited. Hormones were off-limits after breast cancer. It became another echo of surviving what had already taken so much from me. One afternoon, curled in pain and unable to stand, I told Daren that I couldn't believe I worked so hard to survive for this. I wondered if maybe survivorship had been wasted on me. *Shouldn't I be celebrating life and loving this body I fought so hard to keep? Am I a disgrace to those who don't get the chance of survivorship?*

When I was unable to find relief from pain without self-medicating in ways I feared would become unhealthy habits, I decided to have surgery, which included a hysterectomy. I chose to let go of one more chapter in my body's long, complicated story.

Two days before surgery, I poured a cup of coffee and sat at my laptop after a morning walk with Barley. Writing became part of the healing routine I'd come to rely on. I wrote not just to document my experience, but to explore what I felt beneath it. Initially, I wrote cautiously, careful not to reveal too much. But over time, writing became a refuge, a place to release what I couldn't always say out loud. On hard mornings, I'd pull an affirmation card and write unfiltered, each word a step closer to connection with my body.

My period had arrived, heavy and painful as usual, saturating overnight pads every hour or two; clearly, my uterus was trying to have the last word. That morning, I told my body what it needed to hear in an honest letter addressed to my uterus, tears running down my face as I typed. Through the pages, I was able to name and welcome the anger and grief I had been feeling about this next loss. I also said goodbye, affirmed my identity as a woman, and put myself back on the path to healing.

My doctor was right. I had stage 4 endometriosis. Endometrial implants had adhered my ovaries to my uterus, and even my bowels. The decision to have surgery felt affirmed, and for the first time, my pain felt truly validated. I was proud of myself for trusting my body's intuition that what I experienced was not, in fact, normal. I began to see that the seeds I'd planted had started to push their way through the soil.

When I reflect on my cancer journey, I return to the image of emerging from the mountains to cross the prairie. Prairies, I've learned, need fire to clear what no longer serves them and make space for new life. After the burn, plants flourish from the ashes, as the soil is fixed with important nutrients. I've come to see my body's ongoing challenges, like endometriosis, as fires in my prairie. They are painful, yes, but they are also clearing the way for growth and beauty I'm only beginning to see.

* * *

It's been nearly eight hours since we arrived at the tattoo shop, and I'm the last one left. One by one, the others' tattoos were revealed, and then they said their goodbyes. The other artists and the event's coordinator have all come to hang out with me and Daren as Natalee puts finishing touches on her art. I don't mind being the last one. It further reinforces my confidence in Natalee's attention to detail, and I know she wants to get it just right for me. Finally, I hear the buzz of Natalee's tattoo gun stop, and I know she's finished. She stands up, shakes her wrists, and smiles proudly.

I'm handed a black shawl with a pink breast cancer ribbon pin on it to cover myself as I sit up. The photographer who's volunteered her time and has been there all day, rushes over to catch my reaction to the big reveal.

I sit up slowly, my lower back stiff from lying on the table most of the day. Everyone gathers around me, and their faces tell me I'm going to love it. I turn to face the large mirror on the wall behind me. Slowly, I let the shawl drop from my shoulders and see the finished artwork on my chest. It takes my breath away. The fine black linework of the zinnias and butterfly, resembling a vintage botanical journal and evoking the beautiful complexity of life, covers both reconstructed breasts, symbolizing my transformation. Emotions flood my body as tears of joy well up in my eyes, and I realize this is the moment of celebration I have longed for. The photographer captures it all, from my messy hair to my smile through the tears. For the first time since my diagnosis, I feel at home in my body. And it is beautiful.

* * *

My breast cancer diagnosis sent me on the journey to wholeness that I didn't realize I needed, because, as is with most life-changing events, we don't know we aren't whole until the pain illuminates the holes that need to be healed. This journey has taught me to embrace all the ways I've felt broken, without judgment. It means allowing myself to feel all the human emotions, including those I've tended to avoid, like anger and grief. It means learning to trust my body and honor its wisdom and resilience.

On my journey, I'm learning to hold the complexities of my body with greater self-compassion and grace. I can have days where I am disappointed that I have to adjust my plans because of my chronic pain *and* be grateful to be alive. I can miss the body I used to have with curves that looked flattering in A-line dresses *and* be proud of the healthier lifestyle choices I've adopted since having cancer. I can grieve the loss of my breasts and my uterus *and* know that not using them to bear and nourish children doesn't make me any less of a woman. I can see a therapist *and* still need antidepressants.

Being able to hold the complexities of my body gives me the strength to hold the complexities of the messy world beyond it. As I lean into them, I hope they help me have greater empathy for others, leading me to deeper connections and more authentic relationships.

The never-ending journey to wholeness is not linear, just as I learned that grief is not linear. It can be ugly and muddy, leaving one impatient and wondering if beauty will ever emerge, much like a prairie in early spring. In his essay, "Spring is Mud and Miracle," teacher, writer, and activist Parker Palmer said, "Before spring becomes beautiful, it's plug-ugly, nothing but mud and muck. I've walked through early spring fields that will suck the boots off your feet, a world so wet and woeful you yearn for the return of snow and ice."

The last five years have changed me, and I cannot be expected to be the same. It would be nice if I didn't need cancer or the fire to fully realize this, but that's out of my control. The best I can do is tend to my body and soul with grace and intention, much like I tend to my zinnia gardens each year, trusting them to bloom in abundance, purpose, and joy.

AUTHOR BIO

Born and raised on Ojibwe land on the shores of Lake Superior, Melissa is a first-generation college student who always worked hard. After dedicating fifteen years as a middle school teacher, she found herself face to face with burnout. She made the difficult choice to step away from the classroom, and she joined a nonprofit that supports educators in creating more belonging in schools. Less than a year into her career transition, and as the world went into the COVID lockdown in March 2020, Melissa was diagnosed with stage 2, HER2-positive, aggressive breast cancer. Amidst layered crises, she underwent chemotherapy, bilateral mastectomies, reconstruction surgeries, and various complications. Since her cancer diagnosis, she's had to navigate continued health challenges. Even so, Melissa continues to say "yes" to healing as she works on trusting her body and embracing what it means to be fully human.

Melissa loves and finds awe in the natural world, especially plants. She often takes lessons from the wisdom plants have to offer. In her free time, she enjoys being outdoors, gardening, volunteering as a Master Gardener, baking, and letting her creativity run wild. She lives on Dakota land in Saint Paul, Minnesota, with her partner Daren and their dog Barley.

LAUREN LOPRIORE

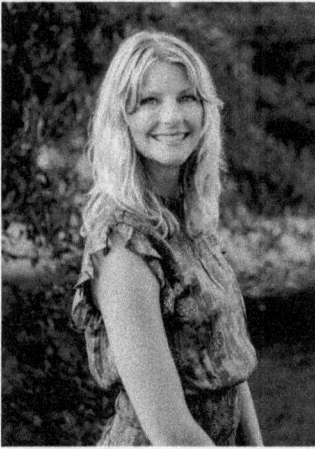

It was a strange, emotional tug-of-war—learning to accept the new me while mourning who I used to be. I started to find the strength I possessed, somewhere under all the armor I had built under the guise of being perfect. All my life I had been hiding in an effort to protect myself, because I was afraid of not belonging—of being rejected from my family, from my husband during this cancer journey, from myself, as I changed and evolved because I couldn't stop it. But the surprising thing about evolution that you didn't choose is that it forces you to either quit or rebuild a new foundation. One that is formed from the blood sweat and tears of a new and stronger self. Vulnerability is a strength I soon learned.

HIDING IN PLAIN SIGHT

"Would you like the photos with your scars?" The New York City boudoir photographer's question hung in the air, almost too intimate for the space we were in. I was about to let myself be seen in a way I hadn't allowed myself to be in years—vulnerable, raw, unguarded, exposed.

I hesitated. For years, my body had been a battlefield, scars mapping out the fight I fought and survived. I stood there, shifting uneasily in my new olive-green silk bra and matching slinky underwear I treated myself to, feeling its coolness against the heat building inside me. I'd never felt comfortable naked—had never learned to love my skin like some do. I had never been the kind of woman who reveled in her body.

And then, I thought back to the day of the surgery—the purple dots marking up my breasts, the coldness of the operating room and the soft hum of machines that would soon take over my body. As I lay there, counting backward from ten, I tried to find some semblance of control, but the truth was, I was being stripped down in a way I couldn't stop. The surgeon's hands would take what they needed, slicing away parts of me. And before I knew it, my chest would no longer be mine in the way it had been. Four slices—parts of me I'd lost forever.

Did I want my scars showing in the photos?

Yes, there were the scars—the physical ones that traced the journey of my survival—but there were others, hidden deeper, in places I hadn't let anyone see. The ones my eyes saw were hard-earned, each one not just a reminder of the battle, but the proof of what I had survived. They weren't a weakness. They were evidence of strength and the courage I hadn't known I had. It was about reclaiming my body, my identity. They were a part of me.

"Yes," I said, my voice a little stronger than I felt. "Yes." I glanced at the other sexy lingerie pieces I had purchased for the shoot and was ready for my show to begin!

The woman staring back at me through the lens wasn't perfect, wasn't unbroken—but she was real. And that, I realized, was enough. I wasn't going to hide anymore. Ready to let the world see me as I was, flaws but standing tall, scars included. I had been stripped down to the studs, and now, I was ready to start building again. Scar by scar. From hair to toe.

Big Apple Vulnerability

It didn't take me long to realize the truth: The Empire State of Mind wasn't the place for me. It was everyone else's dream, but I could never quite fit into it. The people I met seemed to have their lives figured out—chasing the kind of success that glittered with fashion, marketing, finance, and theater. I was just trying to figure out how to pay my rent and buy myself an overpriced salad once a week. Every day felt like a race I didn't even know how to start, let alone win. I couldn't fail,

I couldn't let my parents down, yet I needed them to accept me for who I was.

But my body knew something I wasn't ready to admit. It knew long before my mind caught up. I made it two years in that city, drowning in a sea of crowded streets and bright lights, until my anxiety started to show its ugly face. The panic attacks came in waves—unpredictable, violent, and crushing. I'd go days without sleep, caught in this cycle of stress, my chest tight with every breath, my mind spinning in a loop of worst-case scenarios. New York, with all its endless noise, became a hot box that toyed with my emotions and trapped me in my thoughts. The more I tried to escape, the more I felt the weight of being stuck—physically, mentally, emotionally.

The subway doors opened and I stepped on, the person next to me brushing my shoulder roughly. *Is this how I travel to work each day?* I wondered as I searched for a place to hold on tight and keep me upright as the train sped up to deliver us to Midtown. Smells of foul body odor punched my senses as I thought about taking the subway to the train at Harlem transporting me to Pelham where I once drove my car to work. The next stop was mine and the doors opened. There was a flood of New Yorkers standing in front of me, waiting for me to get off so they could get on. As I attempted to exit, I was met with another shove from an oncoming passenger. My immediate response was "Oh, I'm so sorry," as they continued past me nearly knocking me over. This was the last time I ever said sorry. My sensitivity started to change from caring to frustrated, a feeling I eventually became disgusted by. The only thing I actually wanted was to be noticed, to be visible. I had been good—kind, generous, soft where it counted. But what had it gotten me? In that city, it felt like kindness was currency no one wanted to trade in. I didn't get anything from being the person I thought I had to be.

Then the anxiety came in like a speeding taxi and railroaded my anonymity by gripping me with very visible bouts of panic and fear.

There were so many decisions to screw up. My nervous system couldn't take it because the city was turning me into someone I didn't like. In order to survive I had to ignore the kind and quiet girl I was, because that is what my life had always required of me in order to survive. I became the stereotypical New Yorker: rude, impatient, and always in a rush. It got to the point where I wanted it all to end. I needed it to end. Not as in my life ending, but as in, I needed to move away, get away, be away from all of this. I had just wanted to take some time to figure out who I wanted to be after college and serve on a quiet island. But now look at me, the sounds, the lights, the people who looked right past me were stripping me until there wasn't much left of the girl that moved there a few years before. I needed to be significant, somewhere, to someone. I was not fine. But I told myself, "You're fine. Get over it."

Despite the hardship and frustrations, I found someone who became significant and to whom I was significant. He heard me, he saw me, he let me be me . . . and all of that made me uncomfortable. I didn't know what it was like to be heard or seen the way Eric saw me. Even with this important connection, it still did not keep the anxiety at bay. I needed calm, quiet, nervous system regulation.

In a moment of sheer desperation, both of us on either side of my studio apartment's bathroom door, backs to each other, panic squeezing the life out of me, I spoke my truth and said I needed to go. I couldn't do this anymore. All the noise, the chaos, the running into doors slamming in my face. I stayed for five more years after that night and prayed for the day I could finally go.

Windy City Resilience

Finally, life brought us to Chicago and I couldn't have been more relieved. We had just gotten married, found a great place to live, and for the first time in seven years, I felt like I could actually breathe. Chicago was walkable but not isolating, and I could actually buy a salad for lunch every day if I wanted to without it costing an arm and a leg. We moved into our floor-to-ceiling windowed apartment overlooking the river. I smiled every time I looked out at that pretty fantastic view. I had paid my dues and the price had been hefty. I had been stripped down to a person I didn't recognize. But life was looking up and I was ready to start living joyfully as the me I wanted to be, instead of just surviving.

Walking the river brought me so much bliss and I was always shocked when my happy smiles were returned by the others on their daily walks. I soon began to start living the way I wanted to, feeling good in my body, in my mind, and moving on after the years of discomfort and finding space in a new environment hoping to make it home.

* * *

Yoga was still new to me when we moved to the Windy City from the Big Apple, but it became a familiar activity that brought me comfort and relief from the anxiety that was starting to surface again. I had discovered yoga while living amongst millions on the island of Manhattan, and embraced it as an escape from the bright lights that poured into my apartment windows at all hours of the night, a respite from the grating sound of sirens that ricocheted off my brick walls at any given time of the day or night. In the beginning, yoga wasn't much of a practice, it was more of a struggle. I could barely hold Chaturanga—falling as I shifted forward, doing my best to lower into a four-limbed staff pose. But I kept going because this was the one thing I didn't want to give up on. I used to give up on things when they got too hard—or when the friend I was doing it with quit. I didn't have the courage, the self-compassion, or the support I felt I needed. No one was standing on the sidelines saying, "You've got this." And sometimes, the frustration won. Yet, movement was a layer I wanted to hang tightly to.

In Chicago, the walk to the yoga studio became part of my spiritual ritual. Our apartment sat in a wind tunnel near the North Branch of the river, and I'd zigzag my way east, weaving through the noisy tourist corridor that felt more like Manhattan than the Midwest. I'd always scan the skyline for the skull logo stamped with El Hefe Super Macho Taqueria—my odd little landmark that told me I was close. Just beyond the thrum of hard rock music and after-work conversations, I'd find the narrow staircase tucked away, leading up to the studio. Climbing those stairs felt like déjà vu—like the old walk-ups in New York where my relationship with yoga had first begun.

But a year later, in the tucked-away Chicago studio, that relationship started to evolve. My experience on the mat shifted, and slowly, the connection I had with my body began to unravel again.

At the end of that summer, I began to feel pain in my chest after class. It was dull at first, then sharp—a stabbing on the side of my right breast. I held it instinctively, trying to soothe the discomfort, and then, as I moved my fingers across my skin, I landed on a firm bulge. It protruded slightly out of my skin. I kept pressing, tracing the area carefully, and then found something else: a small, pea-sized knot tucked under my right arm.

"What the hell is this?" I said aloud, though no one was around to hear.

Had I pulled a muscle? Strained something? It didn't feel like the tension lumps I'd had in my neck for years—those were familiar and I knew they were stress-related. This felt different. But still, I pushed the concern away. My body had been a map of mysterious aches and pains for nearly a decade—IBS, acid reflux, inexplicable leg pain. Surely this was just another blip in the landscape of my anxiety-filled body.

But the next yoga class left me in even more pain. The soreness in my right breast and underarm was back again and impossible to ignore. The lumps were still there. I walked home, alone, mind racing.

What could you even pull in your breast? I wondered. And then, the inevitable dark cloud descended. *Could it be breast cancer?* I stepped into the apartment, unsure of how to share what I was feeling—literally and figuratively. Finally, I approached my husband.

"I feel a lump on my breast. And another one under my right arm. It is painful and it moves," I told him, my voice calm, but concerned.

I didn't want to go down the Dr. Google hole, but my need to know how serious this could possibly be, and what I could do to help it heal, won out. After talking with my husband, I called my mom and told her, "I've started feeling this lump on my breast and under my right arm pit. What do you think it could be?" I massaged the lump and took note of the fact that it moved from side to side. "Google says breast cancer lumps don't move and don't hurt so it can't be cancer, right?" My mom assured me that it most likely wasn't. My intuition told me that I should call my doctor just to have it checked out. Google left me mostly with breast cancer links, but I wasn't willing to accept that cancer could even be an option. I needed an expert opinion.

"You're too young for cancer," the nurse practitioner explained to me after I had answered her question about my age. "Twenty-nine years old is just simply too young, so I wouldn't be concerned. I'll write you an order for an ultrasound."

The waiting room was a sea of fifty-five and over patients. I was the youngest by thirty years. As I looked around and calculated my odds, my figuring was interrupted by a nurse who called me back for an ultrasound. I tried to lay calmly, but all I could think was: *What if it is cancer? How long have these lumps been here?* The examiner excused herself and returned quickly, explaining that the doctor was going to come in and take a look. I immediately searched her face for a sign.

"I'm thinking this is not good," I said.

She calmly held my gaze and replied without skipping a beat, "Let's just wait until the doctor is able to come in."

The doctor reconfirmed my fears when he sent me in for a mammogram right then. I searched my brain for what that meant. *Aren't mammograms for women over fifty? Why would I need to have this test done?* I walked to the next room, where a nurse cupped my breast onto a cold metal platform and then proceeded to smoosh it like a waffle machine mushing the batter down. It hurt, but I am a lot stronger than I knew and was able to get through it. They asked me to wait. There was always so much waiting. I took a seat on the small couch in the corner and settled in for my results. It felt like forever had passed by the time the doctor came in to tell me, "We think it's breast cancer." Tears were already forming in the corners of my eyes and trickling down my cheeks, as I reached for the tissue box. My husband had wanted to come with me, and now, I wish I had let him. I needed him now, more than ever. I called him and he said he was on his way. My body was not fine. I headed into the biopsy room so they could remove three chunks of my breast to be tested.

"I've seen these cases a lot. You are young and you will get through this," the nurse told me with a reassuring pat on my shoulder. My husband walked in just in time to give me a big squeeze.

It only took a day for the doctor to call with the results: It was breast cancer. I broke down in my husband's arms as I let the news sink in. I have cancer. I still get uneasy and emotional when I think about that day. High up, on the twelfth floor overlooking the river, having no idea what was ahead. I was twenty-nine years old with a triple positive, HER2-positive breast cancer with a genetic predisposition diagnosis. Immediately following the news, a hollow feeling of loneliness whooshed in and came over me. I felt alone. I didn't know anyone else my age who had experienced cancer. Other than my grade school teacher, my grandmother had been diagnosed with breast cancer at a young age, and then experienced a recurrence when I was in high school. She was young, yes, but she was also no longer living.

Being left alone with my thoughts left me feeling sad, and my mind was confused which only heightened my anxiety. I just couldn't think straight. After a long and eerily quiet weekend, my week began with a list of appointments that would reorganize my life for the next year; the oncologist, breast surgeon, breast reconstruction surgeon, radiologist, fertility navigator, and fertility counselor would all become regular rotations on my calendar. One of the first questions the oncologist asked was if I had a family history of breast cancer. I shared what I knew of my grandmother's metastatic diagnosis. Sitting with me in the tiny oncology patient room was my husband Eric, mom, and aunt. My aunt joined me as a second mother figure, someone I grew up with and was very close to. There was silence for some time until my aunt (my mom's sister, my grandma's daughter) spoke up and said, "I had breast cancer." I was already in shock, but now this news only brought me into more of a confused state. "What?" *How did I not know? I would be fine*, I told myself. *I had to be fine.*

* * *

The following days were spent learning about skin sparing, breast implants, in vitro fertilization, estrogen, how chemotherapy destroyed ovaries, the viability of eggs, whether biological children would be possible, and what to do with our embryos. I met with the breast surgeon, breast reconstruction surgeon, the fertility physician, and the fertility councilor all within the span of two days. My brain hurt from trying to absorb these new terms, translate medical jargon, and comprehend the multitude of ways my body would be stripped of what made me a woman. My stomach turned at the news that my perfect blond hair would fall out. My throat closed up when they explained how my breasts would be removed. And finally, my heart went numb as I absorbed the information about how much toxins my insides would be filled with, so much poison that my chances of having children were drastically reduced. After a lifetime of striving for perfection, it seemed perfectly ironic to consider how completely and utterly imperfect I was going to be when this was all over.

I moved through my days paralyzed, like a deer caught in the headlights of a great big cosmic dump truck headed straight for me. Thank goodness I had a scribe with me because it all sounded just how my life felt in that moment, like my life's song had been playing beautifully, and then cancer scratched the heck out of the pleasantness of my life. The heaviness I felt left me without any spirit. I had very little energy, just enough to walk myself in and out of each appointment. The breast surgeon and reconstruction surgeon were serious and matter of fact. As we sat around the circular table, a sketch of two sets of breasts was drawn on the back of the green info sheet laid out in front of us with the words "skin sparing" and "nipple sparing" written above. One had nipples with a dotted line around each and the other had two lines straight through the center. Because of the BReast CAncer (BRCA) gene and where the cancer started, removing the nipple was his recommendation.

The reconstruction visual was a computer screen of women with breasts of various sizes and shapes. Who knew there were so many sizes and shapes? The only discussion regarding reconstruction of my breasts was moving forward with implants. I wasn't a candidate for DIEP flap—a reconstruction using my own lower belly tissue—and the option of staying "flat" was never brought up by the plastic surgeon. He wanted to ensure that my body would be transformed back to "normal." I had no idea what my options really were; how could I know what would be best for me down the road? I was solely reliant on my medical team and had only their recommendations to follow.

If losing my breasts wasn't enough, the words "You will lose your hair" sent chills down my spine, causing the knots in my stomach to tighten. Of all the side effects, this one felt the most personal, the most jarring. Even more problematic than the loss of my breasts. For as long as I could remember, I had been a blond-haired girl—naturally. Shoulder-length hair with bangs, usually curled under in a way that suited me. I'd grown out the bangs, cut them, grown my hair long, trimmed it short again. It was more than just hair. It was who I was.

I asked my stylist to cut it all off. The pixie cut was the most drastic change I'd ever made. It looked nice—but I couldn't enjoy it. It marked the beginning of everything that would come next. I was slowly being stripped down by each strand that fell to the ground.

I decided to make this drastic hair cut move right before my husband's birthday. Anxious, no terrified, I didn't know how he would react. He loved my hair just as much as I did, pulled back and off my face. *What a birthday present*, I thought bitterly as I studied myself in the mirror. He was hearing not only did his wife have cancer, but now the woman he had fallen in love with would be changing in ways neither of us could control. *Would he still think I was beautiful? Would he still see me for who I really was?*

When my stylist turned the chair around, I stared at my reflection as tears welled up in my eyes and rolled down my cheeks. The cape was still draped over me like a shroud, but what I saw staring back felt unfamiliar. A breeze from the salon's vent grazed the back of my neck and I shivered, not from cold, but from vulnerability. Butterflies churned in my stomach and then I realized, it actually looked . . . nice. I wanted to enjoy it, however it wasn't just a haircut, it was a signal to start all the pain and uncertainty that was to come next. That's why the tears kept falling. When I got to the front door, there was no turning back. I opened it, self-conscious in my shortened hair. My husband looked at me and smiled. "Look at you, beautiful . . . I love it!" I couldn't make eye contact with him. No matter how hard I wanted to believe him, I just couldn't. At least not yet. How could I? I wanted to feel beautiful. But all I felt was grief. For the woman I had been before this moment. For the one who had spent years letting her hair grow past her shoulders—long and soft, a veil I could hide behind. That hair had been more than hair. It had been my identity. I was being stripped. Not just of hair. Not just of breasts. But of everything I'd used to define myself. Everything I'd used to protect myself.

* * *

I had been dreading this day, but because of the timeline of hair usually beginning to fall out two to four weeks after you start treatment, I knew it was time. The owner of an intimate and personal boutique near where I grew up, gently brought the buzzer to my scalp and, within moments, took away every last piece of hair—leaving only a thin, fuzzy layer behind. Just a few days later, I began to notice small strands of hair left behind on my pillow. *It's happening!* Was all I could think as I stared at my hair strewn across my pillow. The real shedding. Watching the patches form even wider on my scalp—those bare, uneven spots— was harder than I could have ever expected.

I will never forget the first morning I went to wash my hair. Well, really my scalp. I lathered the shampoo I used for my long hair in between my hands and was still expecting to work it into the hair that once fell down my back. I found myself shocked, all over again, at the feeling of my hands gliding over my scalp. All I could see was the cherry-red skin tag on the back of my head, and suddenly, I realized just how utterly exposed I was. I broke down into sobs as the hot water poured over me, mixing in with my tears. *Would I be okay?*

The first time I did acupuncture was the day after I received my second chemotherapy treatment. It wasn't until right before the second round that I was introduced, better late than never. I don't recall the introduction, but when I was informed that it could help with the side effects caused by chemotherapy I told them to sign me up. Nausea, yes, vomiting, yes, pain, yes, anxiety, yes, and bowel issues, yes! I made appointments every three weeks at the integrative medicine office where I saw my primary care doctor. And it *worked*. The second round wasn't as brutal as the first. My body, which had felt like it was unraveling, began to hold itself together again with the help of the thin filiform needles. I wasn't into woo-woo things at the time, but after the diagnosis I had just received and the side effects I already experienced, I was willing to try anything.

My hair started to come back—dark and curly, nothing like the blonde strands I had always known. As the tiny dark specks began to break through the surface, I would catch my reflection and have to remind myself to breathe slowly. *Who was I now?* Each time I looked in the mirror, I saw someone new. Someone who had been irrevocably changed. But instead of resisting it, I decided to lean in. I began to experiment—rocking all sorts of styles as my hair slowly returned, growing in centimeter by centimeter. As I walked through the city with my freshly grown, cropped curls, strangers would stop me to say how great my short hair looked. I often found myself doubting their words, brushing them off as pity disguised as praise. *They're just being nice*, I'd think. *They feel sorry for me. They meant well.* I could see their kindness. But every compliment landed me in a complicated place. It was hard to say "thank you," because deep down I hadn't chosen this look. It wasn't a bold style decision or a trendy cut—it was the aftermath of trying not to die.

It took a long time for my hair to grow past my ears, but along the way, something unexpected happened. By embracing each new stage—every awkward length, every curl that sprang in a different direction—I began to see the woman underneath it all. I started to see that I wasn't just my blond hair. I wasn't the face with makeup. I wasn't the clothes I wore. I was so much more.

It was a strange, emotional tug-of-war—learning to accept the new me while mourning who I used to be. I started to find the strength I possessed, somewhere under all the armor I had built under the guise of being perfect. All my life I had been hiding in an effort to protect myself, because I was afraid of not belonging—of being rejected from my family, from my husband during this cancer journey, from myself, as I changed and evolved because I couldn't stop it. But the surprising thing about evolution that you didn't choose is that it forces you to either quit or rebuild a new foundation. One that is formed from the blood sweat and tears of a new and stronger self. Vulnerability *is a strength* I soon learned.

I had been brave. I had gone away to school, moved across the country, lived with a family I didn't know, moved into Manhattan, all while struggling with anxiety and depression. I survived job loss, financial insecurity, and lost friendships. I had cut my teeth on adulthood in the Big City and somehow, came out the other side, all grown up. If I could make it there, I could make it anywhere, I decided. The same girl was within me, she just looked different, and I was fine with that. Instead of focusing on what I had lost, I intentionally focused on the green eyes staring back at me in the mirror. Like muscle memory, I began noticing the familiar shape of my nose, the height of my cheekbones and reminding myself, it's just hair, they are just breasts that I wasn't attached to, it was just a form that I hid my true self in. I would be fine, I had to be.

Everywhere I looked, I saw reminders of what I didn't have. Friends were starting families, and my reproductive system had been shut down. There would be no baby bump photos, no natural conception—only a series of losses and complicated grief.

"Your ovaries will most likely not function properly after chemotherapy." Words that were like a dagger being jabbed at my heart. We wanted children some day. How would this happen if we couldn't naturally conceive? This was all I knew, having children the natural way. I was losing the reproductive capacity to grow our family with biological beings of our own. In vitro fertilization was an option we were told about. We discussed retrieving eggs, pairing them with my husband's sperm, freezing them in a tank, and when we were ready they would be available. I froze sitting in the counselors chair as she discussed that sometimes you get a lot of eggs and sometimes you don't so as to be prepared. I was already losing my chest and now more of my lady parts were being slowly removed like a game of operation.

And should I stop hormone therapy (tamoxifen), that was blocking the effects of estrogen in my breasts' tissue to prevent the growth of any more cancer cells so I could carry our children? Would we look into adoption? What would the surrogacy process look like? I was reminded of my imperfection, how much my body had been through and the loss that I encountered in less than twelve months. I wasn't ready to stop the one thing in my mind that would help prevent my cancer from coming back so surrogacy and adoption became our family planning options. The looks my parents gave me when we shared surrogacy would be the route we would take left me feeling less than perfect. I was not fine. They would eventually come around to it, but I will still remember the note my dad sent after their visit, "Mom and I are sorry for the response or lack thereof that we gave you about your news. It's new for us and we didn't know how to respond." This left me shoving that response down, suppressing the grief I had and the feelings of how broken and unfit I felt. I felt like the black sheep feeling judged and baa-ed at by the fluffy white ones.

The loss of carrying my own child broke my heart more than I realized. We were making up for lost time as we weren't getting any younger and treatment had taken a year of our lives away. Surrogacy was an option where we could use our genetics to create a beautiful being. Even with a surrogate, our path to parenthood was paved with grief—failed transfers, donor eggs, a miscarriage. Every try reopened the wound. My ovarian function, most likely sending me into premature menopause as well, was reduced to nothing. I was sick to my stomach after the blood tests showed my children would not be even a sliver of me. It's still a struggle to this day to know that when we share the story of how our children came to be in our lives that I am only sitting on the sidelines feeling the loss that I had no control over.

Our daughter would finally arrive bringing us joy and happiness. We were told we should just appreciate that we had our daughter, but we knew we wanted another child. Using the same surrogate, we tried again with our freshly generated embryos. I would experience loss unlike ever before. My hair, my breasts, this was nothing compared to the loss of embryo transfers and a miscarriage. Over three years we were brought to tears and heartache each failed transfer—there were two and one miscarriage. From being told that you have a heartbeat at the eight-week appointment that could join the other energized heartbeat you fought so hard to have to being completely crushed when, at eleven weeks, the heartbeat is no longer heard. We lost a little girl. The grieving was real, but hidden to all around us. It was painful. It hurt down right to my very core. I was a good person, kind, generous, caring, fun (or so I thought), and I was a survivor.

Why was this struggle so real? No one understood the grief we were experiencing. It was a gut punch when my sister, who was also diagnosed with the BRCA genetic predisposition diagnosis and had a prophylactic mastectomy, announced she was pregnant. I was supposed to be having my second child via surrogate at that time. It was hard for me to look at anyone with a pregnant belly, but it was even more of a wound that would be difficult to heal knowing that she had been given the opportunity to reduce her risk, move forward with family planning, and go on living. I was then expected to be present. I was told I was fine and I had to get over the loss I had experienced. I was her big sister.

After the transition back into the office after working from home for the year of treatment didn't go as I had hoped, I chose to make a job change. I was not fine with the energy of the environment I had been away from for so long. I felt different, the space felt different, my colleagues were different around me. But, I couldn't leave my job then, and I couldn't leave now. However, I made the decision to work part-time. I was only able to give part of me to the job while the other part was still suffering at home. It turns out my body knew something again was not right, just like when I needed to leave NYC, and the day of the gala I had been planning with the woman's board, it called quits on me. I had an overwhelming surge of intense fear, my heart racing and my breath short. I felt a rush of doom and, ultimately, this panic attack would keep me in bed for the remainder of the day. Tears streamed down my face while I heard my husband call my boss to tell him I would not be in attendance. I again was not fine.

Finding The Light

The panic attack was the turning point. I was not fine and I didn't have to get over it. I began to learn that it was okay to not be fine, to grief the losses, but also be grateful for my life. Fine is what I would say to my husband when I didn't want to talk about all that was eating away at me inside. Knowing me so well, he knew I was far from fine, that I was hurting and had so much to say. I had spent so long not speaking up and asking for help because I was rejected by the people who were supposed to support me. How could I let it all out now? Cancer had stripped me down to the studs. I was meant to build myself up again from the foundation as Lauren, the survivor, the loyal partner, the mother, the light.

My newborn baby girl named Matilda, meaning mighty in battle, slept upstairs while I started typing up my story. It became the blog Liv & Let—a supportive hub for thrivers, fighters, and caregivers. It was time to focus and prioritize myself, but also share my experience to provide support for others who would have cancer enter their life. Not only did I fill the site with blog posts I had written, but guest blog posts, a calendar of programs and events, a library of resources and product recommendations. Adventure travel with other survivors, meditation, cancer programs supporting survivors through art and education, holistic therapy and services and solo retreats were ways that I started to show care for myself. I had to share these supportive opportunities with other warriors like me. I hoped it would be different for them, but what if they were in a situation like me where support showed up for the first few months and then slowly disappeared when treatment was over and I looked good; no one ever asking how I felt on the inside.

I took the invitation to become visible in my own way. Cancer peeled me open, but the experience and the person I was becoming walked into the healing space that was just waiting for me with the positive energy and the ears to listen. Instead of just pushing through life as I had before, I became more gentle with myself. Having compassion for the twenty-nine-year-old whose world was turned upside down helps me give myself grace when negative energy fills my space and emotions rise up within. I've learned that the emotions aren't simply negative feelings but rather signals providing insights into our needs, desires, and unmet needs. Embracing the process of mindfulness and self-reflection has been a positive step towards greater understanding of myself and having greater self-awareness. Just as I have with myself, being with others, like my daughter, with gentleness gives them the comfort and permission to open up when they are ready. This has helped me to be more empathetic, adding to the sensitivity I already have inside me.

I finally recognized that I was not "fine" when I reacted in a negative way when my daughter fell for the first time and wasn't perfect (in my eyes). This became a starting point for self-compassion, seeking specialized support, and wanting to ensure my children knew they could fall, make mistakes, use their voice, and be their truest self.

I later asked why I didn't know about my aunt's cancer and why I didn't see more family and friends. It was made known that they thought I knew and they believed I wanted it to just be my husband and I in the boxing ring. They knew I would get through it, I was strong, I was told. They believed I would be fine and I would get through cancer. I didn't ask for help much, but when I did suggest company for dinner after chemotherapy, traffic or school trumped time with me. I had enough to focus on and didn't always know what I needed. I wasn't conditioned to ask for help around the house, laundry, or cooking. I was visible, but invisible at the same time to family and friends. Cancer forced me to be visible, but there were still people who found it difficult to show up. Maybe because they couldn't.

The year I completed my Herceptin treatment, my husband and I formed a team of family and friends—Lauren's Posse—for the Lurie Cancer Survivors' Celebration Walk & 5K. We walked in the pack of purple and grey shirts along Lake Michigan, celebrating life. At one point we walked past my survivor spotlight photo—"Attitude is everything" I had written under my face. I had my face out there for all to see with only an inch of hair back on my head. I had breast cancer and I was participating in the survivor celebration walk. Was this how I really felt or what I thought I had to say? All that I wanted was to be seen as the zebra I was, but many times I hid in the mix of stripes to feel accepted. I had a good attitude about it all, but years later I'd realize that the good attitude wasn't going to help me rise out of the experience. There were still wounds to heal from, including the loss of my team members walking beside me each and every year until it was just me and my husband walking. Processing and resolving the deep wounds didn't happen automatically.

* * *

In the final frame, after I was finally able to let loose, the photographer, also a survivor, draped me in a pink flowing cloak. I spun around the room, barefoot and unguarded, letting the cloak swirl around me like joy made visible. The image captured more than a moment; it revealed a black sheep no longer hiding behind the blur. A woman who had walked through pain, and was growing comfortable not fitting in the frame others had chosen. Cancer forced me to refocus, but I was the one who chose to keep the lens honest. I was building a new and stronger composition—one rooted in purpose, shaped by self-love, and sharpened by the kind of clarity that only comes when you stop pretending to be fine and be who you really are.

AUTHOR BIO

Lauren Lopriore is a breast cancer thriver, wellness advocate, and mother to two who turned her personal journey with stage 3 triple-positive breast cancer into a mission-driven movement for emotional and practical support.

Diagnosed at age twenty-nine, she founded Liv & Let and Giv Shoppe to ensure no one feels alone during the challenges of cancer and to educate others on health and wellness.

Lauren actively works to break the stigma around difficult health conversations, empower caregivers with tools for emotional resilience, and advocate for compassionate, science-backed wellness practices.

She serves on Northwestern's Adolescent & Young Adult (AYA) cancer program advocacy group BOARD39, advising programs and amplifying cancer support for young adults. She also serves on the community council for Share Our Spare, supporting the awareness, education, and advocacy the organization provides for families living in poverty and the agencies that serve them.

To connect with Lauren visit livandlet.com or givshoppe.com

MARCIE JOHNSON

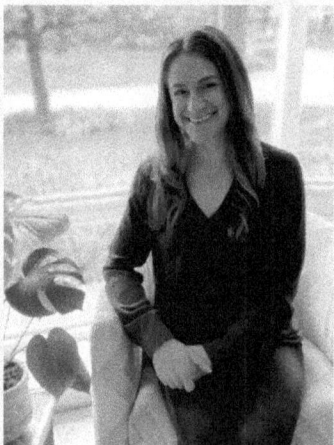

Being diagnosed with breast cancer felt as though I was living out my worst childhood nightmare. It was as if God, or the universe, or whatever higher power may exist, was conducting an elaborate exposure therapy specially designed just for me. It felt like a cruel and surreal twist. I was facing my ultimate fear, the thing I had spent years learning to manage but never truly believing would happen to me. The only way forward from here was through. I would either drown or rise above.

EXPOSURE THERAPY

A Mother's Story of Fear and Fierce Love

The Moment Everything Changed, I Thought of Him

I'm telling this story for him. It's important that I make sure he will always have a piece of me. I need him to understand how deeply he is loved. He must know that he does, and always will, matter to me. I offer these words to him now, in case life doesn't give me the chance later. This chapter is me reaching across time to give him what I've lived, what I've felt. It is a transference of love.

My story could start in many different places, and like most stories, it is not linear. A life is made up of the stringing together of moments. Every moment is affected by every other one, in ways we may not even ever understand. So then, each moment could be the beginning or could be the end.

For me, though, this story begins with the moment my life changed forever. The funny thing about a life changing moment is that all the little ones that come before it are so ordinary. Waking up (always a good start), morning hugs and kisses with my seventeen-month-old son RJ, getting dressed and ready for the day. A sore breast from my biopsy two days before. That was a bit out of the ordinary—but by no means extraordinary.

Fridays were always a race out the gate. Kissing my sweet little guy's silky head, I expressed gratitude to his nanny as I headed out for the day. I chased down toast with coffee from my travel mug and checked the speedometer to remind myself to slow down as I neared W Lake Avenue. I had already been caught by the speed camera and gotten a ticket earlier in the month.

Arriving at work, right on time, I hauled my stuff into my office and settled in at my desk. I was working three part-time jobs—and I felt like a performer spinning all of those little plates on sticks. One job was in private practice as a clinical psychologist, one was teaching psychological assessment to doctoral students at a local university, and one was doing community engagement work. On this day, I was at the university clinic where I shared an office space with another faculty member. I was only in one day a week, so the office was really his and I was just borrowing it for the day I taught my class. The walls were bare, a bland off-white, and there were no windows; but I was used to it. I had been a graduate student for seven years and spent far too much time in broom closets that were generously referred to as "offices."

After checking my email and reviewing some student reports, I closed the door to the office to hop on a virtual call for my community engagement work. The call was held weekly and was a platform to discuss a wide range of health topics and answer health related questions from the community. Our core group consisted of a critical care pulmonary specialist, a pharmacist, and me, a mental health provider. All angles were covered. Each week, about forty community members from different walks of life—community health workers, spiritual leaders, teachers, older adults, to name a few—gathered to listen to an expert present on a relevant topic. That morning, I was listening to a renowned infectious disease doctor share about the risks of infectious diseases in vulnerable populations. My mind began to wander, and I aimlessly reached for my phone. As if on autopilot, I tapped on my email and watched as some new messages updated on the screen. A message about new lab results from my medical chart caught my eye and my thoughts pivoted from infectious diseases to my biopsy earlier in the week. Cavalier as it may seem now, I was not too worried. Yes, I am BRCA1 positive, meaning I have a genetic mutation that puts me at higher risk to develop a variety of cancers including breast cancer. Yes, I had felt a lump in my breast a few months ago, which prompted the need for follow up tests. But I had received a clean mammogram result just nine months before. And my saving grace: I was only thirty-two years old.

As the community call carried on in the background, I opened my medical chart to verify that all was well. My eyes searched quickly for the results and landed on a column that was labeled: Final Diagnosis.

I dropped down to the next line to read:

Breast, left, 12 o'clock, 2 cm from the nipple, ultrasound-guided core needle biopsy - Invasive ductal carcinoma, grade 3 (poorly-differentiated)

Everything in my sight went to tunnel vision. As the room around me blurred and the walls started to close in, I closed my laptop quickly before anyone online could see me pass out or start to hyperventilate. My heart raced as though I was running from an axe murderer, hell bent on taking me down. With shaking hands and a buzzing in my brain, I took a screenshot of the test results and sent the photo to my husband, who is a doctor. I watched as the message was delivered and immediately called him.

"Hey, what's up?" he answered.

"Did you see my message?" I asked, using everything I had in me to keep my voice steady.

"No, I'm in surgery. Why?" he replied.

"I think I have breast cancer," I gasped, gulping back tears.

"What? Why? Calm down, honey, calm down . . ." His voice sounded so far away.

There was no calming down. I was in full panic, gasping for air, sweat pooling at my hairline and in my armpits. My thoughts were racing so quickly that it felt as though I couldn't catch any of them. The blank walls of that borrowed office were closing in on me as my world and life as I knew it started to crumble all around me. Finally, I caught onto one of the thoughts whirling in my brain and it was simply: I am going to die. "I'm going to die!" I shouted into the phone. "I'm not going to be here to see RJ grow up!"

My Journey to Him

Getting pregnant was a difficult journey. It began in 2019, a year into a marriage that was strong and filled with love. We decided to start trying to have a baby, knowing that it could take time. Both my husband and I are in the healthcare field, and we knew that an uncomplicated pregnancy and delivery is not as typical as most of us grow up believing. Like every cancer story, every fertility story is unique.

Nonetheless, with a sense of excitement, we looked forward to growing our family and began trying. You never really think it will be you who experiences the hard stuff. To our delight, we were pregnant within a few months. Six weeks into the pregnancy, however, I started to bleed, and, after various tests, I was diagnosed with a molar pregnancy.

The "mole" (our name for the tumor growing in my uterus) was as bad as it sounds. Basically, when my egg and my husband's sperm met, rather than forming a zygote, they formed a tumor made of abnormal placental tissue that, if left to its own devices, would invade my uterus and my body like cancer and kill me. The tumor expressed high levels of human chorionic gonadotropin (hCG), the pregnancy hormone that peaks in the first trimester and is responsible for the early joys of pregnancy, like nausea and fatigue. I was the sickest I had ever been in my life. The nausea and fatigue were crushing, and I could not get out of bed. I actually think my brain sort of went into shutdown mode, protecting me from the discomfort, and preventing memories from forming and sticking.

Getting rid of the mole required two surgical procedures. The first procedure was a routine dilation and curettage (D&C). After the first procedure, however, some abnormal cells must have been left behind and the mole started growing back . . . so back to the procedure suite I went. I underwent a more aggressive D&C, which did the trick. My bloodwork was monitored weekly until my hCG levels reached zero, indicating that there was no tumor left. After this, I was monitored monthly for six months, and my husband and I were forbidden to get pregnant.

When the six-month pregnancy embargo lifted, we got back to it and about nine months later, I became pregnant again. Shortly into my second pregnancy, however, I started bleeding and miscarried. The miscarriage was devastating. I was so mad at my body for failing me, yet again. Up until the molar pregnancy, I had trusted my body. I believed that it could do what it was supposed to do. But after the mole, that trust began to waver. My body had failed to follow the pregnancy playbook I had imagined it would, and I was left bewildered by the strange and unexpected turn of events. I did not know how to make sense of what had happened. At first, I chalked it up to bad luck and tried to move past it. But when the second miscarriage came, it was harder to explain away. I was left with an empty womb—and a growing, painful understanding of how my body could betray me.

Follow-up tests showed scar tissue in my uterus, likely related to the aggressive procedures required to eradicate the mole, and I was referred to a specialty clinic. I ended up needing another procedure to address the scar tissue—the physician went in, cleared out the scarring, and placed a balloon in my uterus, which I then walked around with for a week. Balloons are so much less festive when they are inside your uterus instead of being used to decorate for a party.

By the fall of 2021, two years after I became pregnant for the first time, I learned I was pregnant again, this time with RJ. As pregnancies go, there were some small bumps along the way. Overall, though, we were blessed with a healthy pregnancy and a delivery that only left my body somewhat in shambles. Having made it to the other side of what felt, at times, like a never-ending journey, we welcomed RJ in the summer of 2022.

Early parenthood was beautifully challenging, as it often is for new parents. It was a huge transition, and we were learning to juggle old roles with new responsibilities. RJ was the most beautiful baby—exactly how nature intended parents to think. He had a head full of blond hair and bright blue eyes. We were amazed by his every move, his every sound. Of course, there were times at three in the morning that his sleep grunts didn't seem so cute. But after trying so long to have a baby, having RJ finally felt like a missing piece of my soul had clicked into place.

The next weeks and months following RJ's arrival were full of many changes. We moved halfway across the country, bought a house, and started new jobs. RJ did not like to sleep, and my husband and I were tired in a way we had never experienced before. There were nights that I was in with RJ every hour, feeding him, rocking him, cuddling him. The fatigue was no joke and some days it felt like we were moving through the day like zombies. Looking back, though, those memories are sweet; life was busy but good. The challenges we faced were temporary. Our little family was strong and looking forward to a bright future.

Family History

"You still have your breasts? You have not had a mastectomy?" the doctor asked with surprise in her voice, studying my chart and then glancing over as if to check that my offending breasts were still truly there.

"I . . . I . . . I'm still breastfeeding," I stammered back in reply.

It was my first appointment with my new primary care physician, and I immediately felt flustered. In the cold sterile room of her office, I felt the heat rising from my neck into my cheeks. I tried to explain. "My understanding was that increased surveillance is recommended ten years pre-onset of the earliest breast cancer diagnosis in the family. No one in my family had breast cancer before their late fifties . . . and I wanted to breastfeed . . ."

She was visibly displeased. I was feeling defensive because I felt she was basically implying that I needed to chop off my boobs right there in the office. I was still breastfeeding RJ, who was only three months old at the time, and it had actually been one of the smoothest parts of motherhood for me. I was like a blue-ribbon dairy cow and felt pride in my ability to produce milk. I was not ready to chop off the "ladies" (as I affectionately liked to call them). I even hoped we would have more children and that I'd breastfeed again in the future. The suggestion to amputate my body felt almost as if my doctor was amputating my vision of the family I planned for and the motherhood I dreamed of. I made it clear that I was not ready to discuss a prophylactic mastectomy. It felt insulting that she could so casually suggest I get rid of the ladies.

"Okay," she replied, "I think you should at the very least start increased surveillance soon and consider a prophylactic mastectomy after you are done having children. With your family history, it is what I'd recommend."

My family is Ashkenazic Jewish and there is a family history of a BRCA1 genetic mutation, which increases the risk of developing breast, ovarian, and other types of cancers. My maternal grandmother had breast cancer in her sixties and eighties and, ultimately, died of metastatic disease at age eighty-seven. It was not until my grandmother's second breast cancer diagnosis that genetic testing was becoming more accessible and her physicians recommended she undergo screening. Results came back positive for a BRCA1 mutation. She shared these results with my mother, aunt, and uncle and encouraged them to get tested as well. My mother was also positive for the BRCA1 mutation and went on to develop breast cancer a few years later. Luckily, knowing her genetic status, she was doing heavy surveillance, and her cancer was found at Stage 0. She underwent a lumpectomy, radiation, and five years of endocrine therapy.

Like any self-respecting Jewish mother, mine immediately pushed me and my siblings to get tested after she learned she was BRCA1 positive. The rule-follower that I am, I got tested at age twenty-six.

The results came back in big, bold, red letters that screamed off the page: RESULT: POSITIVE - CLINICALLY SIGNIFICANT MUTATION IDENTIFIED. It probably should have felt like a bigger moment, but honestly, it didn't. It wasn't great news, sure, but it wasn't surprising either. I kind of just shrugged, made a mental note to follow up with my doctor, and went on about my day.

I discussed surveillance and prophylactic options with my medical providers at the time. I was young but even then hoped to have kids at some point and be able to breastfeed, if possible. Given that no one in my family had been diagnosed with breast cancer before their late fifties and everyone had kept their boobs, my providers felt it was reasonable to do surveillance and then revisit any possible prophylactic surgeries after I was done having children. The most aggressive surveillance protocol was to alternate between a mammogram and an MRI with contrast every six months. However, I was concerned about such frequent exposure to X-rays and contrast for so many years. As I understood it, aggressive surveillance should start at least ten years prior to the earliest onset of disease in a family. For me, that would put me somewhere in my forties, when regular surveillance is recommended for all women anyway. So, I elected to do minimally invasive surveillance of the ovaries and do regular breast checks myself.

My new doctor clearly disagreed with my surveillance plan and insisted that I have a mammogram in a few months, even if I was still breastfeeding, and that I get an MRI with contrast after I finished breastfeeding. Willing to compromise, I agreed to this new plan. A few months later, I followed through on my end of the agreement and had a mammogram. To my relief, the results came back clear.

Fast forward six months, and by now RJ was a year old and I had weaned him off the boob. Before motherhood, I knew my boobs pretty well—their weight, their shape, the way they changed with the ebb and flow of hormones. Motherhood had already transformed them, stretching and deflating them in ways I could not have imagined. So, when I felt the lump, like a smooth marble had been placed beneath my skin, I told myself it was just another leftover change caused by nursing. Another shift in texture, another trick of hormones.

I run nervous, though, so had my husband check it out, just to be sure. He was not overly concerned. The lump wasn't unyielding the way the model boob with a pretend tumor felt in health class. I could sort of move the lump around with my fingers; shift it up and down, back and forth. We decided it probably was not much to worry about, and I took to monitoring it for the next few months.

At my annual physical two months later, my doctor asked if I had any specific concerns that day. I mentioned that I was having some joint stiffness in one finger and some wrist pain. She examined my finger and wrist and put in an order for blood work just to rule out anything serious. As she was getting ready to leave the room, I remembered the lump on my chest and, almost as an afterthought, asked if she could feel it. With icy fingers, she palpated around my breasts and chest, leaving a trail of goosebumps in her fingers' wake. After the exam, she concluded that the lump felt cystic to her. However, given my BRCA1 status, she wanted me to have an MRI with contrast anyway, as part of increased surveillance.

The results of the MRI showed abnormal lesions in the left breast (where I could feel the lump) and in the right breast (which I could not even feel), warranting further follow-up. A few days later I found myself back at the doctor's office for an ultrasound and biopsy.

Life Can Be Hard—And We Can Do Hard Things

The results of that biopsy were like an earthquake that shook my life to the core, cracking the foundation of my reality and sending tremors through every part of my life. The world I knew split open, exposing a terrifying new landscape I never planned to navigate. Over the next eleven months, my body would endure an unrelenting assault—surgery, fertility treatment, chemotherapy, and radiation. It was to be a crusade of cutting, poisoning, and burning, all in the name of healing.

In the first weeks following my diagnosis, panic attacks seized me night after night, gripping my chest in their vice, leaving me breathless, shaking, and in tears. I could barely eat. I could hardly sleep. The thought *I won't see my baby grow up* haunted me at every moment. And in the quietest, darkest pauses, I came face to face with something I had spent my whole life outrunning—my own mortality.

Humans are biologically motivated to stay alive, so it makes sense that death scares most of us. I am no exception. According to family lore, at three years old I sat my grandmother down for a philosophical discussion about death. I wondered about what happens when a person dies. Where do they go? What happens next? Death is the ultimate uncertainty and uncertainty is terrifying, especially for an anxious brain like mine.

As a child, the scariest thing I could imagine was cancer—because to me, that meant death. A family at my school had a son who was diagnosed with brain cancer, and after surgery, he was left with significant mental and physical impairments. The fear of cancer, illness, and disability took root in me, developing into intrusive thoughts that consumed my mind and disrupted my daily life. I spent hours performing compulsive, ritualistic behaviors, desperate to "erase" the bad thoughts about cancer, to convince myself I was safe, that I wouldn't get sick, become disabled, or die. The shame of these obsessions and compulsions weighed heavily on me—I hated that these thoughts existed at all, and even more that they had such control over me. I was only seven or eight at the time so did not totally understand or have the words for what was going on in my mind. It was a scary, exhausting cycle.

Fortunately, my parents noticed the changes in me and got me into therapy. I worked with a child psychologist who specialized in exposure therapy, a form of cognitive behavioral therapy designed to help manage obsessive-compulsive symptoms. Together, we created a hierarchy of feared situations, and I gradually exposed myself to each one, all while resisting the urge to alleviate my discomfort through compulsive behaviors, like washing my hands or showering. The principle behind exposure therapy with response prevention is that, through repeated exposure over time, the brain learns that a feared thought or situation is not inherently dangerous. By facing the fear and allowing time to process it, the intensity of the fear gradually diminishes.

One of my exposure exercises involved a headscarf that my therapist brought in from a friend of his who had breast cancer. He explained that his friend had lost her hair and used this very scarf to cover her bald head. At eight years old, I found the sight of chemotherapy-related baldness deeply frightening—it was one of the most visible and unsettling signs of illness and reminders of death. My assignment was to hold the scarf and rub it on my body. I was to sit with the anxiety it triggered, resisting the urge to flee or perform any compulsive behavior to manage the discomfort.

The exercise was excruciating. The fear manifested as physical discomfort on my skin. I felt as if I had a layer of grime coating my body and all I wanted to do was wash it off. Everything in me screamed to do something to "protect" myself from the "contagion" (even though

I logically understood you cannot catch cancer) but I did not. Instead, I rated my level of anxiety on a scale from zero to ten and watched as the anxiety peaked and then slowly declined.

Over the years, I became skilled at managing my anxiety. Whenever scary thoughts of cancer or disability wandered into my mind, I learned to notice them, endure the temporary discomfort, and watch as their power over me weakened. I learned to weigh the evidence in support of or against the likelihood that I really did have cancer. I learned to calm my mind by reassuring myself that there was little evidence to support most of my worries. Anxiety is like a false alarm. It is the brain sending a warning signal that you are in danger, even when there is no real threat. With practice, I became an expert at coping with these false alarms and learned to navigate the anxiety around the *possibility* of having cancer. Once the possibility became a reality, however, all bets were off. This was no longer a drill.

Being diagnosed with breast cancer felt as though I was living out my worst childhood nightmare. It was as if God, or the universe, or whatever higher power may exist, was conducting an elaborate exposure therapy specially designed just for me. It felt like a cruel and surreal twist. I was facing my ultimate fear, the thing I had spent years learning to manage but never truly believing would happen to me. The only way forward from here was through. I would either drown or rise above.

When Life Gets Heavy, Let Laughter and Love Lighten the Load

I knew it was coming. After two rounds of The Red Devil, a chemotherapy blend of Adriamycin and Cytoxan—a bright red cocktail injected into my body every other week—I couldn't move my head without clumps of hair literally dropping from my head and landing on the playroom floor, gathering on my pillow, or piling up in the shower drain. Every single time I saw a clump, my heart raced, and I checked my reflection to see where it had detached from my head this time. It was as if every single part of my body was screaming: *This is really happening! You have cancer!*

My thirty-third birthday was approaching and instead of sitting like a ghost of myself in the darkness of my bedroom and wishing away the day, I decided to take back control. I contacted Lucy, the hairstylist I had worked with earlier in the month to choose a wig, and told her I thought it was time to shave my head. Lucy is an amazing human, herself a cancer survivor. After being diagnosed with stage 4 blood cancer that had spread to her bones at age thirty-four, Lucy underwent a year of chemotherapy and fought tooth and nail to survive. Her doctors told her she would not see her son, who was four years old at the time, grow up. They told her that even if she beat this round of the cancer, it would inevitably come back. But Lucy refused to accept that. She vowed that if she survived, she would dedicate her career to helping other people going through cancer get wigs. She understood the impact of hair loss on self-esteem, confidence, and morale. Now, forty years later, Lucy continues to help those with chemotherapy related hair loss find hair prosthetics that make them feel a bit more like themselves, pre-diagnosis. And her cancer has never returned.

Lucy had me come to the salon so she could shave my head for me. My mom and sister came with me. They were not going to let me go through this alone, on my birthday no less. I've always been curious how I would look with dark hair and a blunt bang but was too scared to ever try it. I'm not a big risk-taker when it comes to appearance. The wig I chose was darker than my natural hair so I could try out the look. "Hey," I thought, "If the universe gives you an opportunity to test out a new look, you might as well take it." Before shaving my head, Lucy cut a bang so that I could see what it looked like too. All I can say is it's a good thing I had not risked it prior.

My sister Ali also experimented with some new looks at my appointment. Lucy had many wigs and other hairpieces at her salon and my sister really leaned into the experience. Ali is a spicy, hilarious, gregarious woman, who can be counted on for a laugh. As Lucy was shaving my head—an experience that I thought would totally gut me—my sister decided to see how she'd look in some new hairstyles. She donned a bang hairpiece, a completely different color than her hair. It looked absurd. But instead of tears of sadness that day, I only cried tears of laughter.

I named my wig Rachel. The name of the style on the box was "Raquel" and I decided Rachel was a better fit for a name for me. For a wig, Rachel looked good. She was chestnut brown and went a little past my shoulders. If I wore a hat over her or a headband on top, she looked pretty realistic. Nothing against her, but I never quite got used to wearing a wig. The pressure of it on my head felt unnatural and gave me a headache if I wore it for too long. And when I caught my reflection in the mirror, it just did not feel like "me."

Luckily, my husband and son hardly noticed whether I was wearing Rachel or just went bald. The first time I showed RJ my bald head, he simply touched it and moved on. I had worried that he'd be scared or cry, but the reality was that he was completely unphased. I was amazed and relieved.

Like father like son, one night when I was giving RJ a bath my husband walked in after a long day of work. I had also worked that day and was wearing a little makeup. But I had taken Rachel off as soon as I got home to be more comfortable. I was kneeling by the bath, face made up, and completely bald. My husband walked in, looked at me, and said, "You look so nice today, honey!" He hadn't even noticed that

I was bald. He just saw me. I could feel the love and gratitude swelling inside of me. Even though I felt different, to my husband and son I remained the same. With or without hair, I was beautiful to them.

Strength Finds Us Rooted in the Present Moment

When people hear my story, they often remark on my "strength" and ask how I "did it." The truth is, how I did it had little to do with strength. I've learned that there is no way to prepare for how you will respond when the whole world starts shaking around you. I think most people would be surprised by their inner drive to keep going, get healthy, and live. Both for themselves and for the people and things that matter to them.

Coping with a cancer diagnosis and battling through active treatment was not easy. The beginning, as my diagnosis and treatment plan unfolded, was particularly hard. There was so much unknown and everything felt off-kilter. Humans are extremely resilient, however, and we adjust to even the hardest of circumstances. We learn ways to protect ourselves and those we love. We laugh so that we don't have to cry. We joke so that everything does not always have to seem so serious. We look for safety and connection when fear and uncertainty scream in our faces.

To be perfectly honest, I'm not totally sure how I've survived the past year and a half and how I continue to survive the fear of recurrence. I used to have a vision of what my future might look like. Of course, I always understood there are no guarantees in life, but for the most part I was generally able to ignore the ever-looming possibility of death. For better or for worse, that all changed with my diagnosis.

In psychology, there is a construct known as *time horizons*, which refers to a person's perception of the remaining time they have left in life. Time horizons influence behavior, goals, and priorities. While individuals with long time horizons tend to prioritize goals that require long-term planning and investments, like getting an education, building a career, and building a social network, those with short time horizons tend to focus on goals that provide emotional satisfaction, like spending time with loved ones and pursuing activities that bring joy.

It makes sense that young people often have long time horizons. A long time horizon allows us to make the sacrifices necessary to build the lives we want. We work grueling hours to get the degree we want, even if it means less time to spend with friends right now. We have babies to create the family we dreamed of, even if it means less sleep right now. We stay at work late so we can get that promotion, even if it means missing bedtime with the babies we wanted so badly. When the time horizon is long, we can push off the present for the good of the future.

For me, being diagnosed with cancer was like getting bitch-slapped by the present moment. With just one medical test result, my time horizon shrunk, and the present moment took on powerful new meaning. The overwhelm sent me into an existential tizzy. The big questions—*What makes life meaningful? How can I live a meaningful life if I am going to die young? How does anyone lead a meaningful life since we all could die at any moment?*—spun inside my head. My brain felt like the ocean during a storm. My thoughts were dark, angry, choppy, swirling. They felt too big to contain within me, heavy, dragging me under the churning waves, as I struggled to come up for air.

Through this chaos, though, came some clarity. The reality is: I cannot control the future. But if I do things that are meaningful to me each day, when I die, I will have lived a meaningful life. I know the saying goes, "The whole is greater than the sum of its parts." But maybe the truth is that the whole being equal to the sum of its parts is enough. No offense, Aristotle.

As I've clawed my way back toward the shore of health and no evidence of disease these last few months, identifying who and what matters most to me and doing things each day that move me toward those people and things has become my life raft. When worries about the future or regret about the past start to pull me down, focusing on the things I can do to live a meaningful day today helps me stay afloat. That's not to say that I don't often take in lungfuls of water. But it's something.

I've identified the things that are meaningful to me to do each day—which I call my "daily nonnegotiables." First, I spend quality time with the people I love. This might look like playing with RJ before school, going to my nieces' sports games, or calling a friend to catch up. Second, I do work that feels meaningful. Maybe this is doing psychotherapy with a client or reviewing a paper. Third, I move my body. I might take the dog for a walk, do a yoga class, or play tennis. And fourth, I participate in leisure activities. I love to read, watch television, and write. Whatever it is that I am doing, knowing that, if I move toward these values each day, the sum of my days will be a meaningful life provides me with great comfort and has fundamentally changed my life.

Night Night, Baby

The night before my bilateral mastectomy, I rocked RJ to sleep as I do every night. Holding his little body in my arms, I nuzzled the back of his neck as I sang to him the medley of songs that conclude his bedtime ritual. The first is a prayer that my mother sang to me when I was a child. It is a Hebrew song that affirms the Jewish faith, declaring the oneness of God. The second and third are songs of love and adoration. With his warm little body snug against my chest, I tried to plant my melody in his heart. I kissed his head, placed him in his crib, and whispered, "Night night, baby. Mommy loves you." I tiptoed out of the room, looking back for one last glimpse of him sleeping.

I walked down the hall to my room and shut the door. I needed to be alone. Voice thick with tears, I recorded myself singing RJ's bedtime songs on my phone. In case things did not go well the next day, I wanted him to have these songs to carry with him. I worried that without time, there might never be a way to instill the values that mattered to me in my son. There might never be a way to teach him the important lessons in life. He might not remember the warmth of my hug, the sweetness of my kisses, or the touch of my skin. I might not have the opportunity to tell him each day that he is loved unconditionally, and that he matters, he is enough. He may not remember how much we laugh together and how I think he is hilarious or that, as a toddler, he thinks I am funny too. I may not be there to celebrate the joys. I might not be there to help him through the tough moments of life, to help him find his strength.

So with whatever time I have, my mission has become to create a love that he can carry with him even if I am not around. This story is for him. To show him he is always on my mind and in my heart. To teach him that he can do hard things. To remind him to laugh and find light, even when life feels dark. And to reassure him that he has an inner strength that will one day surprise him.

My grandmother always told me to carry her love with me, and this is what I hope to leave my baby as well. I hope my love is transferred into the fibers of his being. That it is something he *feels* no matter what. That it keeps him safe and protects him. That it is imprinted on his soul the way he is imprinted on mine.

AUTHOR BIO

Marcie Johnson, PhD, is a thirty-four-year-old mom, wife, daughter, sister, friend, psychologist, and breast cancer survivor. As a licensed clinical psychologist, Marcie works with people across the lifespan to support mental health and resilience. In October 2023, at age thirty-two, she was diagnosed with invasive ductal carcinoma (hormone positive), an unexpected challenge as a young woman, new mom, and early career psychologist. Marcie underwent eleven months of treatment, including a double mastectomy, five months of chemotherapy, and thirty rounds of radiation, and is currently in maintenance treatment. Her personal journey with breast cancer has deepened her understanding of vulnerability, suffering, strength, and the human ability to heal.

LEANNE KALLEMEYN

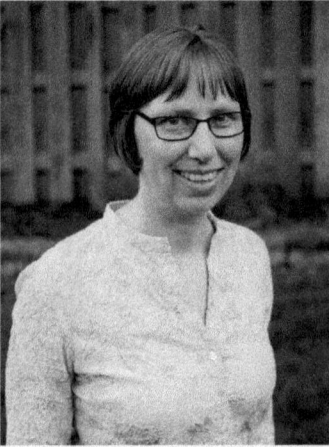

Resiliency was not continuing to do what I had always done. That was insanity. Anne Lamott's description of hope resonated with me: "Hope begins in the dark, the stubborn hope that if you just show up and try to do the right thing, the dawn will come. You wait and watch and work: you don't give up." This decision, to take a break and figure out what I really and truly wanted, was pivotal in my healing journey, because I was respecting and caring for myself. I had learned to listen to my inner voice.

LISTENING TO MY INNER VOICE

Sometimes life comes crashing down, providing opportunities to recreate wholeness, restore joy, and renew hope. This reality becomes very clear as I find myself at a two-day writing retreat, sponsored by the University I work for. As I walk footpaths cleared out around a large pond, I spook white-detailed deer and observe geese navigating the melting ice, stopping to take in the early spring sound of birds singing. The colors are still that of winter, bland, bare tree branches meet the heavy gray clouds, and root down into the brown grass, but an inhale of the fresh air is moist and warm and reminds me that, indeed, life is able to renew. I am here to work on this memoir and publications for a faculty promotion, a goal I had let go of four years earlier when I was diagnosed with breast cancer.

Each night after dinner together, faculty gather in small groups to share. Tonight's question is "What is one thing that is currently *life-giving in your work?*" The question itself is laden with the infallible truth that our work in academia is life-giving. To admit otherwise would be an audacious, counter cultural act. I mull over what I will share as I am going to be last. We happen to all be women of various ages and backgrounds. As I listen to their life-giving stories, I realize that their experiences involve moments when they gave life to students—some created structures to provide clinical experiences and meaningful class assignments, and others addressed how they handled overt racism in class and supported a student dealing with an oppressive situation. Many even mentioned how taxing this work was for them, and they were reconciling how it was still life-giving. It is life-giving to others. That is what we do and how we think as women.

When it is my turn, I speak my truth rather than something aligned with the normalized narratives I have heard. Four years ago, I would have been anxious and completely censored something misaligned with norms, but at this moment, surprisingly, I feel a sense of courage and excitement. I explain that I was on medical leave a few years previously, and I started a practice of daily journaling. My prompt was exactly like the one we were given today. I wanted to discover what was actually life-giving for me. What I learned from that journal practice surprised me; my work was not life-giving, but rather, going for a walk, immersing myself in nature filled me full of life. Eating a good meal with people who cared about me and who I cared about, cultivating social connections—that gave me life. I discovered that it was in these simple moments that I felt complete, and in return, I was able to work. "If I have to choose something life-giving in my work, it would be this retreat." I finished my share and looked around the circle, still amazed at what I said and curious how long it would take to break the silence. One of the women in the group finally responded with, "Wow. That is an amazing perspective." She paused. "I am curious what led you to start journaling." I take a deep breath. I am willing to share, if they want to understand.

* * *

It's a few weeks before Christmas and I am meeting with my medical oncologist for the first time. It's been just a few days since my biopsy results came back and as she gathered my history, she asked if I had felt anything different in my breast before I had found the lump a few weeks ago. I shook my head emphatically and replied with certainty, "Nothing." I explained that in my annual visit with my primary care provider in August, no issues had emerged in the exam or my labs.

Later I remembered how the leaves were changing at the end of September, how the air, while warm, was beginning to hint that a change in seasons was upon us. We had been staying in a cabin nestled on a bay of Lake Michigan for a long and quiet weekend. It was a much needed break from our busy suburban Chicago life. As a professor navigating COVID, I was chronically exhausted, overworked, and overdue for rest, even before the pandemic started. And so was my thirteen-year-old daughter Leah, who was in the midst of a flare of symptoms from a chronic illness. My husband Jeff, Leah, and her eleven-year-old brother Joshua, canoed the bay, floating around on calm waters, admiring lily pads, catching whitefish, anticipating how much we would enjoy them for dinner. In the evenings, we played games and I laughed until my dimples hurt, engaging in friendly competition. We watched the sun rise and set, admiring the stars that popped out a few at a time, lighting up the dark night sky.

On our third morning, I woke up with the sun, rather than my husband's obnoxious alarm, and while it was relaxing to stay in bed, I felt unproductive. I remembered that I was almost due for a breast exam, which I aimed to do monthly with my cycle but also wasn't religious about it. At forty-two years old, I had a couple routine mammograms with no concerns and no family history of breast cancer, so when I had gotten a letter, reminding me to schedule one during the lockdown, I decided to delay it. It seemed extra important to do a self-exam. As I walked my fingers around the fleshy part of my breast, I felt the usual lumpiness that comes with heterogeneous dense breast tissue. Usually, I could palm my breast with one hand, but this time I couldn't quite do that because it was enlarged. I sighed with the realization that not only was weight gain going to my hips, but apparently to my breasts as well? When I gently used two fingers and felt carefully over each breast, there was a spot in the top middle of the left side that I went over multiple times. *It feels different.* I thought for a minute. I pressed my fingers down gently. *No, it doesn't feel different.* I raised my hand and tried again. I couldn't make up my mind. I made a mental note to check it again in a few days. A couple mornings later, my period started which relieved my concerns, but I also noticed my breasts stayed enlarged. *It must be weight gain,* I decided. *I have got to figure out a way to fit in exercise.*

On a Sunday night in November, almost two months after our long relaxing weekend, I noticed a lump in that same spot, as it changed the natural contour of my breast when I reached my arm back into the sleeve of my pajamas. Immediately, feelings of dismay washed over me, but I managed to rationalize with myself not to worry before I had something to worry about as I fell asleep.

A few weeks later, I found myself emotionally numb as I spent hours in the women's health center at our local hospital, waiting for my diagnostic mammogram and subsequent ultrasound. I had been forewarned that the process would take hours. I brought work along, as I couldn't just sit in the waiting room at this point in the semester. My to-do list would not get done even if I worked a full day. Although I couldn't identify it at the moment, I was completely disengaged and disembodied from the procedure. I couldn't lean into the feelings of fear and anxiety. My work kept me detached. Since I tend to be anxious, in the days leading up to the mammogram, I spent extensive energy rationalizing that I could not worry until I had more evidence.

Hours later, the words of the radiologist after she read all the images stayed with me. She explained that I didn't have one lump, but a cluster of several lumps highly suspicious of cancer, including one small lump in a lymph node in my armpit. She looked at me with such sincerity and tried to assure me, "This diagnostic mammogram is the first step and we will be with you every step of the way." Those words were the only ones that got through my emotional numbness as the reality of the situation started sinking in fast.

By the time I made it to my car, I was in hysterics. This new reality initiated an emotional thawing as I was overwhelmed with sadness and grief. *With all I have done to create a beautiful life for myself and my family, how did this happen?* When Leah was three weeks old, we relocated to the Chicago suburbs so Jeff could start his new job, and I started my tenure-track position months later. Jeff and I had each other, but we did not know anyone when we arrived. Living in the suburbs, I felt more disconnected from others than I ever had in my life. My job was also isolating as the intent was to prove my worth through independent scholarship. I was grateful for so many positive life events that I neglected the stressors my apparently "good life" created. I hadn't taken time to be honest with how alone I felt. I had lost touch with what brought joy in life, being grateful for simply waking up and being alive each morning. As a working mom, I chose to just keep going round and round, as if living life on a hamster wheel. And now, I felt mentally and emotionally whiplashed from being blindsided by life. In that moment I allowed myself to feel how overwhelmed I had been for years.

I returned my husband's multiple texts and calls. He listened to my hysteria from the other end of the phone. I could hear in his voice his deep concern for me as he offered to come pick me up so I would not have to drive home alone. "No, no, I'm fine to get home," I said, and then hung up the phone. He was already working and supervising two kids in e-school. *How could I ask him to do one more thing?* I sat in the driver's seat, alone again, weeping for as long as I needed to before I felt I could drive myself safely home.

Jeff and I went for a walk when I arrived home. The fresh air and his hand in mine helped soothe me. *In all our twenty-one years of marriage, when was the last time we went for a long walk, holding hands and conversing?* I wondered. He remained calm, emphasizing that we would deal with it together one step at a time. He needed to get back to work, and I didn't trust myself to be alone with my racing thoughts. I called my mom, the only other person I told about the lump. I kept crying out in desperation over the phone, "What am I going to do? How do we tell the kids? What if the cancer is advanced already? How will I manage treatments with everything else?" My mom, realizing quickly that I was spiraling, switched from empathy to advisory. "Leanne, this is not something you can figure out and solve on your own. Lots of people are going to offer you help. Don't you dare be independent and not accept it." My mom knew me well. I am the oldest, graduated valedictorian of my high school class, worked to support my way through college, married my high school sweetheart, and then we both proceeded to complete our PhDs together, celebrating my dissertation defense with a cake that said, "Congratulations, Dr. Mom," announcing to friends and family our exciting news. And now after living my dreams for thirteen years, my cake has been smashed.

Nine long days later on a Friday afternoon, Jeff and I got the call with biopsy results that made the diagnosis official. Yes, it was malignant invasive ductal carcinoma. The "good" news was that it was estrogen and progesterone positive and likely HER2-negative, meaning it would involve less treatments than other types. That night, after the kids were in bed, Jeff and I sat on our living room couch, his arm around me, protective, as my head rested on his shoulder. "How did this happen? Why is this happening to me? What are we going to do?" I asked over and over, like a broken record version of my normally assured and levelheaded self. He listened and held me close as I sobbed into his chest and continued to ramble.

Within a few weeks, I started chemotherapy. Due to the restrictions around COVID, I had to go into my infusions alone, just like the diagnostic mammogram. Plenty of people sent texts of love and encouragement and I settled into a routine of calling my sister while my body was pumped with drugs to counter the unintended side effects followed by the toxins proven to kill breast cancer. Hours after the infusion was complete, I stopped in the restroom on my way out. My crimson red urine suggested major concerns, but the nurse assured me that was normal due to the drug nicknamed "The Red Devil." Somehow, I managed to drive myself fifteen minutes home, alone.

My mom, who lived a half-day drive away, was part of our COVID bubble. She came to stay with us, carrying out daily household tasks and helping care for our kids. As the rounds of chemo carried on, she stayed for more days, as it took longer for me to nurse back my strength to complete daily tasks.

I considered going on a medical leave, but I was already on an approved 50 percent time research leave. I was told most faculty keep on working during chemo. *How can that be?* I wondered, but I had no energy to address these institutional barriers. Even on days when I had no energy for laundry, I could lay on the couch, reading and writing. Some normalcy felt like a healthy distraction since so much of my life and routines had been drastically interrupted. I was used to being the stalwart supporter offering help to others. It felt foreign to think of myself otherwise, so I needed something I and others still deemed "productive." *Could caring for myself really be considered a productive activity?* Besides, simple tasks like eating, peeing, and pooping repeatedly stirred up worries and concerns, and some days took all the energy I could muster to complete. I could only handle small doses of anxiety, grief, and sadness at a time, and work was a perfect distraction.

People connected me with fellow breast cancer survivors that they knew, and these women warmly accepted me into an amazing sisterhood none of us ever wanted to be a part of. My friend Katie asked if she could share my diagnosis with her mom. A few days later I got this note in the mail.

Dear Leanne,

Katie shared with me your recent diagnosis of breast cancer. I just felt that I needed to write and encourage you. Twenty-nine years ago—this month—I was diagnosed. I had four children in four different schools—college, high school, middle school (Katie), and preschool. I remember struggling and wondering how I could manage chemo and surgery. God brought so many people into my life to help me through this difficult journey. I know he will do the same for you. I am praying for you. Journaling was extremely helpful for me. It helped me to express my feelings, document appointments, and keep track of highs and lows. Best of all, I can look back when I reread them and see God's hand in all of it. When I was diagnosed, I prayed that God would allow me to see all my children graduate from college. Well, he blessed me with seeing all of our children marry in the Lord and give us eleven grandchildren. His goodness goes way beyond our imagination . . .

Love, Kaye

Tears streamed down my face. Kaye's story exceeded what I could even imagine. I was so appreciative of the support my mom provided that next to my gratitude and joys, my journal was filled with grief and fear about whether I would be alive for Leah and Joshua when they were grown. Kaye's story gave me seeds for hope. As the rounds of chemotherapy went on, I was so exhausted and desperately wanted to live a long life that I realized accepting help from others was my only option. I was starting to accept that I was worthy of all of this goodness that others gave me, and I did not need to work to prove my worthiness.

With the fatigue and all the side effects from chemotherapy, I had no choice other than to focus on caring for myself and relying on others. I looked forward to my kids coming out of their rooms on e-learning breaks to check on me. "Can I get you anything, Mom?" They would refill my water bottle, bring me medicine, and warm up food for me to eat. I noticed how much joy it brought them to care for me. *Why had I not given them more opportunities to experience this joy?* I had been so concerned about setting an example of working hard and giving to others, but now realized it was also important to model receiving help.

I gratefully accepted help from friends, family, church members, and work colleagues. They mailed and left care packages on our porch for months—meals, cards, flowers, journals, body care products, gift cards, ginger candies and tea, homemade blankets, knitted hats and socks. *Could reaching out and helping us be a way they filled their pandemic void? Could I really be helping others by allowing them to help me?* Oddly, being in a COVID bubble with four people, I still felt connected to so many people, more people than before my treatments.

When friends asked me what it was like to go through chemo-therapy, I explained that I realized I needed to take care of myself the same way I took care of my kids as infants. After an infusion I would put what was left of my energy into creating new routines that revolved around self-care: sleeping, eating, hydrating, peeing, and pooping. When I could, I would leave a little space for tummy time (I did pilates), socialization, and play. *When was the last time I prioritized taking care of myself all day long for multiple days in a row?* As difficult as chemotherapy was, it felt good to have a reason to prioritize my health and well-being, something that I neglected doing for years. If I wanted to be alive for my kids, I needed to take care of myself. And yet, I grieved not being able to care for my own family by doing basic tasks, like washing the dishes or doing laundry. *Had I ever imagined that I would grieve doing those tasks?*

On the long, dark nights when I could not sleep because my mind raced with fears or from steroids taken to prevent side effects, or possibly both, I laid on the couch journaling my gratitude, with only God as my witness. Although I hesitated for weeks, I eventually read *The Book of Joy: Lasting Happiness in a Changing World* based on conversations between Desmund Tutu and the Dalai Lama, which a student sent me. I found much solace in their thoughts that "There is no joy without sorrow, that in fact it is the pain, the suffering that allows us to experience and appreciate joy . . . true joy is a way of being, not a fleeting emotion." My dad suffered from post-traumatic stress disorder, anxiety, and depression, so from childhood I was familiar with life shattering to pieces and the possibilities of rebirth. Oddly, knowing how much I was suffering brought me comfort to experience fully life's joys—a morning bowel movement, new flavor for my water, my kids choosing not to argue, sunshine, colorful head scarf tied with a new twist, support from Jeff, my mom and so many, and gaining some energy back after another round of chemo. Practicing joy and gratitude were like muscles that had atrophied during the constant hustle of my day-to-day life before my diagnosis. I had not exercised them much prior to cancer, but just like you never really forget how to ride a bike, my muscle memory kicked in. This practice of gratitude helped me calm my fears and find rest.

A couple months later, just over a year into the COVID pandemic, I had finished my eight rounds of chemotherapy. Joshua and Leah had been back to full-time, in-person school, utilizing social distancing practices, for three weeks. The rest of the world was starting to open up, but I still could not join it. My mastectomy was scheduled for Monday, and on the Friday morning before, Joshua came out of his room, face flushed, wearing a look of deep concern. "I don't feel well. I think I have a fever," he said.

For months, I had planned for this exact scenario. I resisted my initial motherly instinct to feel his forehead and soothe him with a hug. I got us both masks, sent him back to his room, and set supplies outside his bedroom door. He checked his own temperature with the digital thermometer and confirmed that he was indeed running a low-grade fever. Through his closed door, I explained the plan for our separate territories. He put on a brave voice, assuring me he could care for himself, which broke my heart. I soothed him with words of comfort, but that was all I could offer. I went to another level of the house, crying in frustration, feeling powerless because I couldn't care for my son. But the truth was, I couldn't risk getting sick three days before my mastectomy. Somehow, I had made it through chemotherapy without getting COVID, and so had the four people in my bubble. I was not afraid of catching COVID, but I was terrified of delaying my scheduled mastectomy, which my surgeon said could worsen my treatment outcomes if not done six to eight weeks after completing chemotherapy.

Jeff and I both went into hypervigilant problem-solving mode, which had been our norm for the last year in the pandemic, complicated by navigating a breast cancer diagnosis and treatment. I took up residence in the basement office, which also served as our guest room. Jeff took on all responsibilities caring for Joshua. He managed to purchase a COVID home testing kit which had just been released to the public. Jeff sent me a text—*positive* was all it said. Joshua had COVID. My heart sank. It felt like learning I had cancer all over again. I knew what was coming, so I was not surprised, and yet the weight of the reality suddenly became physically palpable. Jeff had been shutting air vents, opening windows, and executing numerous strategies to prevent spread. I could hear him walk down the stairs into the basement. I came out of the office, staying on one side of our family room while he remained on the other. We were both wearing masks. He was in tears and overwhelmed, just as much as I was.

"I just want to give you a hug. I need a hug." He sobbed across the space that had been such a place of comfort to our family. I, too, was sobbing uncontrollably, and replied by holding one arm outstretched as if to push him away and one hand to my heart, "You *can't*. We *can't* hug. I *cannot* take that risk. I want to hug you, too, but I *can't*." We both wept on either side of what felt like an enormous divide that left a gaping hole between us. This emptiness was so familiar, after all the treatments I had done alone. Those sobs snapped us out of our frantic efforts to fix the situation—the reality was, there was nothing more we could do.

I had planned to spend Saturday preparing spaces in the house with supplies where I would recover from my mastectomy. And of course, the day before my scheduled surgery happened to be Mother's Day. The irony was not lost on me at all. All I had asked for was some quality time to be together as a family. I had envisioned last opportunities to lay intimately with Jeff before my body was permanently changed. I had imagined how the day would play out, that was a vision that was keeping me going. But again, life had other plans.

Those two days of presurgery isolation gave me an opportunity to turn inward—I didn't have to. I could have spent the entire forty-eight hours ruminating on anxious thoughts spiraling out of control or distracting myself with a numbing activity like scrolling on social media. But instead, I leaned into the silence and the solitude, and I chose hope, the hope Kaye gave me of living a long, full life to be present with my children and their children for decades to come. *Was there anything else worth choosing at this moment?* I couldn't fully articulate it then, but I was starting to realize that hope, like joy, is not so much a belief but a way of being and living. In this moment, even when I had strength to help others, I couldn't while isolating. The only person I could care for was me and doing so brought hope.

Much like the nights early in my diagnosis, my fears were ever present, keeping me awake. I oscillated between fear that I would catch COVID and not be able to have the surgery, and grief over losing my breast. Unlike those initial nights when I let the fear run rampant and grow uncontrollably like a wildfire in my mind that spread through my entire body, I used a prayer journal my friend Katie gave me. I wrote down each fear. When I articulated them on a page, it was as if they had boundaries, a finiteness, and could no longer run rampant in my mind. *Why are you allowing this to happen? Where are you in the midst of my suffering? I need to take care of my family and I have so much important work to do, why are you taking that from me?* I found it was easier to release them. I knew a calm state was a healing state and that my remaining tumor could grow in chaos and fear. More than anything, I wanted to be healed. I breathed in and let the air out. I said a breath prayer that became etched on my heart from guided meditations I streamed countless times during my treatments based on Psalm 16:11.

(Deep breath in) "In your presence

(Deep breath out) there is fullness of joy;"

Over and over until I reached a state of meditation.

That Saturday, I seized the opportunity that can only come from a beautiful spring day. I went for a walk around a small lake near our house. As I made my way around, I reflected on how we had intentionally bought our home near trails so we could enjoy this nature. The irony that it was only during recovery from chemo that I had finally found the time to routinely use these trails was not lost on me. Feeling alone, I called my mom. We cried together, as we had so many times in the last months. Having COVID in our house days before my mastectomy was such an unfair burden to carry. As she had faithfully done, she asked what support Jeff and I needed from her.

On some past Mother's Days I would have been thrilled to have a day to myself, where Jeff took full responsibility to care for a sick kid and made me meals I could eat in peace. But this Mother's Day was different. My heart longed to be with my family, to hug and laugh with them, savoring everything about their presence. I let everyone know we could celebrate another day. The closest togetherness time we had was some social distancing in our backyard, with Joshua joining our conversation through his opened second-story bedroom window. Since this was just another Sunday and I was hoping to have surgery the next day, I attempted to tidy up the office. I replaced piles of paper with clothes Jeff gathered for me. I repurposed a filing cabinet for a nightstand and moved a chair by the window. I had not planned to recover from surgery next to my filing cabinets and bookshelves, the space I associated with work, not healing.

Monday morning dawned, and I was on edge for many reasons, but mostly because I was still waiting for a call from my surgeon's office. About an hour before I was to arrive at the hospital, my phone rang. Jeff and I, once again, stood across each other on our opposite sides of the family room as I took the call. They confirmed my surgery could proceed. Our masks hid our elation and we had to resist the urge to embrace again. I never would have imagined in all the weeks leading up to surgery that I would feel such relief to be heading to the hospital to have my breast removed. Amputating a breast, an intimate part of my body that nourished my kids and brought Jeff and I pleasure, was not anything I was ever going to be ready to do. With cancer there are no good options, just bad and worse ones.

Another bad option I chose was to drive myself to the hospital, again, alone. It was the only option to isolate from COVID. Even though Jeff and my mom expressed concerns, I assured them I could do it. *How would it be different than driving myself for chemotherapy?* Even though I could do the route on automatic pilot, it was different. As I placed two hands on the steering wheel, I would have rather had one gently holding my breast, saying goodbye. The realities of the loss filled my thoughts. I could only focus on what was in front of me—mastectomy. I had no attention left for the rearview and sideview mirrors. I was grateful for a long red light when I could touch my breast, but then the tears and grief started to flow and shutting them off when the light turned green was jolting.

I managed to arrive safely at the scheduled nine o'clock. Surgery was scheduled for one o'clock, but there was much preparation needed, which fostered familiar feelings of disembodiment. The hospital staff were skilled, carefully following protocol. *Yes, due to chemo I am now allergic to adhesive—no tape or Band-Aids. Yes, I have high blood pressure* and take medication. *No, I am not pregnant, but I can pee in a cup to prove it. Yes, the lump is in the left breast. Yes, I am keeping the right breast.* I had become accustomed to these impersonal protocols to ensure I received "quality" care, as all appointments for the last five months had been me having to advocate for myself in the midst of hospital protocols. It put me in a state of alertness. Whenever possible, I played guided meditations on my phone to calm my nervous system, and not surprisingly, a nurse witnessed my blood pressure drop.

I learned after surgery that in addition to my breast, they did find cancer remaining in axillary nodes and had to remove some. I laid in the hospital room alone. *But was I alone?* I felt God's presence. Despite what I had been through that day, my whole being—heart, soul and mind—were overflowing with joy and hope. I was experiencing pure elation. I knew with confidence my body was free of cancer. *How was it possible to feel this way when I had been filled with so much grief and fear hours ago?* At that moment, I realized that was not even a question worth asking. Instead I beamed with a huge smile revealing both dimples and basked in the positive emotions I was experiencing. I had never imagined feeling this way after surgery. Maybe it was the effects of the pain medications, but that night I felt God's presence, an assurance of healing. I was not alone. In the absence of fear, there was nothing calm about these exuberant, positive emotions. The surgeon had shared with Jeff and I that she anticipated she removed the tumors with clear margins. We would know for sure in a couple of weeks after biopsy results came back. I did not need a biopsy result to know that the cancer was gone. I felt it in every cancer-free cell of my body. I was filled with joy and hope.

As I was recovering from my mastectomy, isolating from my family, and no longer working part-time, I was finally in a space where

I could be authentically honest with myself. I was a cancer survivor. If I was to remain a cancer survivor, I needed to understand how I got in this predicament in the first place. *Why did I get cancer? What could I have done to prevent it?* I wrote in my journal and the following thoughts came out:

> *For many years, I have known that commuting downtown and teaching in the evenings is not promoting a healthy lifestyle for me. I have thought about quitting, but I also love what I do. When I started my research leave in fall 2020, I was burned out professionally. I opened myself to new directions and a few months later I had a cancer diagnosis . . . after my oncology appointment today I felt more convinced that my future direction will not be at the university.*

I finished my seven weeks of radiation treatments, an extra precaution to prevent a recurrence, two weeks before the start of the new school year. The rest of the world had been transitioning back to normalcy due to COVID vaccine access for months. I had no evidence of disease, and my oncology treatment team was confidently communicating "go live your life." My family was ready to put this chapter behind us. My energy had returned and I could manage daily tasks again. My mom was no longer coming for extended stays. Everyone around me was resuming normal routines, and now it seemed to be my turn to join them. *But what was normal? What was I returning too? How could I go through this experience and simply return to the way life was before I was diagnosed or before the pandemic?* On the eve of my last radiation treatment, I wrote in my journal:

When I started this journey, I looked toward this day as the one that I was waiting for, the one that would give me my life back. And it will. But I didn't expect to be so worried about the future, endocrine therapy, restoring my health, reoccurrence, returning to work full-time and multi-tasking.

During treatment, I had a clear, focused goal: to make it through treatment and then show no evidence of disease. And I had succeeded. *But now what?* There is nothing like becoming a cancer survivor thrust into medically-induced menopause in the midst of a global pandemic in your forties to set off a midlife crisis. On the outside I tried to maintain and return to who I was before my life had turned upside down, but I knew this no longer matched what I felt on the inside. While my medical team prepared me for getting through treatments, no one had prepared me for the recovery that I needed after my survival.

This became glaringly obvious when I was getting out of the shower one morning and noticed an unexplained red rash and my immediate response was overwhelming anxiety. In an effort to soothe me, Jeff shared several logical causes for the rash and assured me I would be fine. Filled with a fierce anger, I screamed at him, "I am not okay! I will not ever be fine! Life is not ever going to be the same again! It can't go back to normal and never will!" He stopped, listened to my rants, and somehow remained calm himself. My main support network—Jeff and my mom—were getting burned out and they were ready to move on. There was no evidence of disease and my follow-up treatment was no longer affecting their daily routine. However, it was still affecting mine. Every morning, while in the shower, I was reminded that I was a cancer survivor. I needed to be around other women who understood that.

I joined a local weekly support group for "young" women with breast cancer. I realized that even though I felt like I was processing emotions during treatment, there were many times that things moved quickly and I had simply done what I needed to do to get through it. Now that there was space and time, I found that I was dealing with a flood of negative emotions and I didn't have anywhere for them to go. On top of all the emotional processing, I was also trying to rebuild my muscle strength, manage side effects from treatments, deal with medically-induced menopause, and prevent lymphedema. I could feel my body's struggle to keep balance when it had been so disrupted—I was battling constipation, low white blood cell counts, and vitamin deficiencies. *Or was my body resisting resuming my life before cancer? Could returning to this lifestyle also mean my cancer recurs? My body appeared to be in-balance when I had cancer, so did it feel out of balance now that there were no tumors to grow? Or were these symptoms all side effects of treatment?* My medical team could not answer these questions either, but I thought they were critical to restoring my health.

I fought for an endoscopy that showed I had a wheat intolerance, likely celiac. When I woke up from the anesthesia, Jeff was there, holding my hand. I wept uncontrollably. I had done all of my cancer treatments without him by my bedside, and now he was physically there. At that moment, I am not sure what was more healing—evidence of my wheat intolerance that providers kept dismissing or creating new memories of medical experiences with loved ones by my side?

I worked with a dietician to make my temporary lifestyle changes permanent, and yet I could not find time to officially clean out and rearrange my entire pantry. Unlike the cancer treatments that appeared temporary, these changes needed to be permanent. I grieved these changes, as did my family, like the ease of a weekend night to just relax, ordering out for pizza and watching a movie.

I also started to see slight swelling in my left arm and feeling sensations of heaviness, which providers also initially dismissed. I wondered, *Could this be lymphedema?* Lymphedema is a chronic condition that can develop as a side effect of surgery. The lymphatic system is responsible for moving lymph fluid through the body and the armpit is like a major city with intersecting interstate highways. Removing lymph nodes meant that some of my highways had literally been removed. Scar tissue also causes damage and blockage in the lymph system like potholes in the Midwest after the winter thaw. I was on high alert and also holding onto hope that I would not develop it.

When my plastic surgeon finally confirmed my suspicions, I experienced a grief process all over again, right at the one year anniversary of finding my lump and breast cancer diagnosis. *Why did this happen? I had done everything I could to prevent lymphedema and it still developed.* But it wasn't my fault. The breast surgeon removed lymph nodes. *Did I really think that I could prevent a cancer recurrence?*

Within weeks, parts of my arm became like one of those stress balls that you can poke with your finger and gradually watch the indent fill back in with fluid. I noticed daily activities caused more swelling—pushing a grocery cart, carrying heavy objects, doing cat and cow stretches on my hands and knees, and watching my son's indoor swim meets. Lymphedema required one to two hours of daily therapy to manually drain the fluid in my arm. It was like watering plants. If I skipped a day, I couldn't make up for it by doing twice as much the next day. I was only months into resuming life and it had been a disaster. *How could I carve out one to two hours a day for the rest of my long life to manage the lymphedema?* But I had to take care of myself. It was not an option to live my life as I did before I was diagnosed with breast cancer; my only option was to create a new life.

On Ash Wednesday 2021, I had DIEP flap breast reconstruction surgery, followed by a six-week recovery with minimal activity. I was forced to give up a lot for Lent—baths, sleeping flat in bed, daily walks and exercise, travel, work, among other things. By this point, I had become a master of restoring my health and I knew I would rise again. Because I was giving up so much, I chose joy and rainbow moments, eating chocolate daily for Lent.

When I reached the end of short-term disability for surgery, I requested an unpaid leave from work for one year. Even though I had physically healed enough to return to work, I was a wreck mentally and emotionally. I wanted time and space to recreate my whole life. Jeff was discouraging me because he was concerned I would not be happy giving up a career that I had worked so hard to create. I wondered, too, but I was convinced that I had to do it. I realized that resiliency was not continuing to persist despite the odds but rather realizing when to stop, to say no, to give up the things that were no longer serving me. If I did not say no to the stressors from my precancer life, I could not say yes to a new life that would remain cancer-free. Resiliency was not continuing to do what I had always done. That was insanity. Anne Lamott's description of hope resonated with me: "Hope begins in the dark, the stubborn hope that if you just show up and try to do the right thing, the dawn will come. You wait and watch and work: you don't give up." This decision, to take a break and figure out what I really and truly wanted, was pivotal in my healing journey, because I was respecting and caring for myself. I had learned to listen to my inner voice. I didn't know it then, but I was becoming a cancer thriver.

I wanted a new life. I wanted it richer and fuller than the original. During Reiki sessions with guided meditations for cancer patients, I sometimes went back to memories of being five years old, running topless and barefoot in the grass in our backyard. None of the neighborhood boys wore tops with their bathing suits, so I didn't think I needed to either while playing in our small, child-sized swimming pool. I had a short, pixy haircut. I moved carefree between the pool, swing, vegetable garden with sprouting plants, and rock garden that surrounded our mulberry tree. The gentle breeze meant I could smell our hedge of lilacs along the back of our yard anywhere I played. These were experiences of pure bliss.

I took cues from my five-year-old self and started living each day in the moment. I went on spontaneous bike rides to nature preserves. I planted tulips and picked dandelions. I even found a mulberry tree on a walk in my neighborhood and stopped to savor fresh berries. I took afternoon naps when I felt tired instead forcing myself to plow through my day. I developed routines for guided meditation that put me in a deep parasympathetic state, something that had been foreign to my body for years. I tried new recipes and traveled to visit family and friends. I devoured books like Parker J. Palmer's *A Hidden Wholeness: The Journey Toward an Undivided Life* and Martha Beck's *The Way of Integrity: Finding the Path to Your True Self*. I journaled about new life insights, deep pain and suffering, gratitude and joy. I cared for my family in ways I couldn't when I was going through treatment, like making Jeff coffee every morning and packing the kids' lunches. Rather than seeing these as chores, they were a daily reminder that I was alive and connected. All the tasks I didn't have time for before cancer, all the mundane moments of a life I had not truly been living, suddenly became the moments I felt most connected to myself, most alive.

I explored my health and developed a whole new understanding of why my body grew tumors. I learned about metabolic rather than genetic theories of cancer. I maintained the thirty-five-plus pounds I lost and found ways to manage side effects from endocrine therapy.

I experimented and expanded my exercise routines, working with a personal trainer. I did elimination diets and wandered grocery stores reading labels and foraging for quality, minimally-processed food. I established relationships with integrative providers as part of my care team. I connected with other women who were breast cancer thrivers, so I could understand what supported their living. I did pelvic floor therapy and had a third surgery to address lymphedema. My primary care physician took me off blood pressure medication. When my oncologist asked how I was doing at a follow-up appointment, I explained, "Except for the medically-induced menopause, I feel like I did when I was in my twenties." We both smiled, assured this was a good sign.

* * *

Today is Mother's Day. For me this day marks four years since I had two breasts. I say a prayer of gratitude to be alive and experience this moment, waking up next to Jeff. I lay on my back, placing my left hand on my heart and my right on my root chakra. I notice the energy in my body. After a few breaths, I move my right hand up through my chakras. With the deep breaths I am delighted to feel my diagram stimulate peristalsis and waves of calm from head to toes. I imagine the honeynut squash pancakes made with my grain-free flour mix, sweetened with hints of cinnamon and vanilla that I'll have for breakfast with a side of eggs over medium, or some salmon.

I could easily fill my day with university work, start to plant our garden as spring is in full bloom, volunteer at church, take care of the mountain of laundry, watch Joshua at his swim meet, and prepare for Leah's high school graduation in a matter of days. All of these tasks matter to me, but first and foremost I am going to prioritize what fills my soul, and I will discover what that is as the day unfolds. Today I will be. I do not need to work toward societal expectations for a full, meaningful life. My value and worth are not linked to my accomplishments. My worth is simply being me. I will live out my hope that my body will no longer grow tumors. Fear was not serving me and I have let it go.

I suppose to many my life looks similar to before my breast cancer diagnosis, but I experienced this radical shift that has only been possible through incremental changes. Some days I catch myself living by others' expectations and societal norms that do not align with my inner voice. Or, I step back on the hamster wheel, running mindlessly. Other days I allow myself to get lost in spiraling, anxious thoughts of recurrence. On these days, I remember to willingly accept the hands of others who reach out to me. I also graciously reach out to myself with permission to step away with inviting embraces of loving kindness. Through the support of many, I have recreated my life, restoring wholeness, joy, and hope. I trust my inner voice.

AUTHOR BIO

Leanne Kallemeyn is a breast cancer thriver. In her daily routine, she loves to journal, meditate and pray, be present with her family, and touch her barefoot to the ground. Activities that make her heart sing include gardening and cooking, biking and hiking, listening to podcasts and nonfiction audiobooks, traveling to new places, watching the sunrise and sunset, and other opportunities to be in nature. Born in western Michigan, she lives in Libertyville, Illinois, with her husband and two teenagers. She is also an associate professor in Research Methodologies within the School of Education at Loyola University Chicago. She volunteers as a host for a Living with Cancer Healing Circle and is an active member of Wildwood Presbyterian Church, where she cofounded the group WildRide to support others with cancer diagnoses.

JACQUELYN VRANICAR

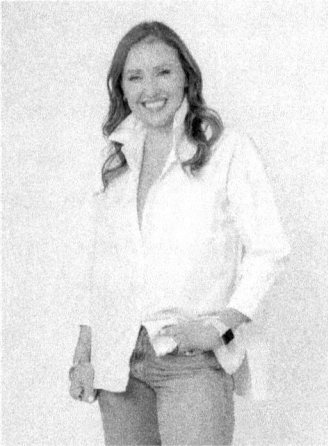

The idea that purpose could rise from something so cruel felt insulting. I paced through denial like a house I refused to leave, slamming doors behind me, unwilling to look at what stood outside. But grief, persistent as breath, kept following me room to room. And somewhere along the way, I stopped fighting long enough to see it: even here, in this broken place, something good could grow.

TURNING PAIN INTO PURPOSE

I am fairly steady, although slow, as I walk toward the end of the driveway. I wince as I feel the pull of my abdominal muscles, the skin tight, thanks to a fresh six-inch incision across my belly—it's only been one week since the surgery. Who knew so many trunk muscles were involved in simply walking down the street? Careful and cautious, I reflect on how quickly things can change; just a few days ago, I was running upwards of five or six miles. The sun feels so warm and welcome on my nearly baby-bottomed bald head, and I notice, funnily enough, that I can feel the tiny new hairs sprouting up all over my scalp because they are growing long enough to sway in the warm May breeze. My husband accompanies me, as this is our current routine—to take an afternoon walk to the bus stop to greet our four children. I'm slowly getting to the end of the driveway when I feel a buzz in my pocket. I pull my phone out and check the caller ID; the screen lights up with the description "U of MN Health."

Seeing this number had once made me stop dead in my tracks. Those first calls had me gripping my phone with a sweaty hand and scrambling to find a private place to take the call—a closet, a bathroom—anywhere I could brace myself for the news that might change our lives irrevocably. But now, those calls had become routine, woven into the fabric of my daily life; they were like background noise. I thought I was on the other side of all of that. I had experienced that first fateful call from the clinic that said I needed to come back for an ultrasound after an initial routine mammogram and the subsequent biopsy. Lying scared on a cold exam table, hot tears pooling in my eyes, and a kind nurse trying to distract me as the biopsy needle was guided into my breast was only a flashback. I had made it through the incredible wait for the devastating news: I had a stage 2, triple-positive breast cancer diagnosis. We had told our two oldest in our bedroom. I can still see it clearly—just twelve and nine at the time, each seated on either side of us, their lanky legs tangled in the comforter, eyes wide with a worry far too heavy for children to bear. Kevin sat beside me, his arm around my shoulders, steady and warm. I had taken a deep breath, the kind you hope fills you with strength, and said the words I never imagined saying to our children: "I have cancer." I had looked into their eyes and immediately followed it with a promise—"But I'm going to be okay." And I had meant it. I had believed it. We spoke softly, carefully, as if raising our voices might make it more real. I watched their expressions flicker between confusion and fear, and I reached for their hands. I needed them to see that I wasn't afraid, even if I was. That moment—so intimate, so raw—had felt like the worst we would face. How could I now take that away? How could I tell them that things had changed, that the promise I made might no longer hold? The guilt settled heavy in my chest, deeper than the diagnosis itself. Still, I had pressed forward—determined to follow the plan, to check every box, to do everything right. I had completed my first surgery successfully, gotten my chemotherapy port placed with only one minor hiccup when all of the prior weeks' emotion and trauma surfaced in the form of me fainting as they tried to start my IV.

I had gone on to endure twelve weeks of chemotherapy and immunotherapy; I knew the taste of saline in the back of my throat as my port was accessed and flushed. I had experienced the physical heartache that came as I stood in the shower and felt clumps of my hair wash down my body as I watched them collect in the drain, and then again, when my husband helped me shave my head. First, into a rocker style mullet to make my kids smile, and hopefully help them cope with the huge shift in their world, and then a week or two later, right down to the scalp.

I was six weeks past my double mastectomy and onto reconstruction at the time of this call. But my body felt as if I had been walking for weeks on end; exhausted from enduring the poison coursing through my body, the pain of sores covering the inside of my mouth, and keeping from buckling under the invisible weight of my diagnosis. All of those experiences had been bearable because I knew there was a light up ahead. I knew I could keep going because there was a checklist I needed to complete to get out of this nightmare and finally be declared cancer-free.

The pang of pulling skin from my newest scar was from removing a benign mass on my liver, and that surgery had gone textbook well. Smooth sailing was ahead of me, I could feel it. There was no reason to be alarmed when the phone rang from the hospital now. I had already done the hard stuff—and I had survived, even if I was banged up and bruised more than a little.

I slide my thumb across the screen to answer, "Hello?" It was more of a statement than a question. "Jacquelyn? This is Dr. Huang." Her voice was hesitant; the halting was barely perceptible, but it caught my attention immediately. "I'm sorry to call you unannounced, but I wanted to talk to you about your pathology results from your liver resection." She stopped again, and then, with a bit of a sigh, she continued, "The results do change your prognosis; five, seven, maybe ten years."

My entire body stopped while the world around me continued on as if nothing had changed. The newly sprouted leaves on the tree-lined streets at the end of our driveway twisted and turned in the spring sun, the approaching bus that was transporting my children hissed to its stop right near our mailbox. The children's laughter that spilled out the door as they ran down the sidewalks to their homes, carefree and unaware, rang hollow in my ears. *Five what? Seven what? What did these numbers mean? The pathology report?* My brain struggled to catch up with my doctor's words. I thought the mass had been removed, and after the PET scan detected it, it didn't "light up" the way cancer does. And even more, what would it matter if it *were* cancer? We had removed it. I had a tender red scar on my side to prove it. I had no idea what my oncologist was referring to as she listed out the years as if they were a timeline of when I should come in for routine check-ins rather than a timeline of what my life expectancy now was.

I don't remember the rest of that call—everything got very blurry and dark. It turns out cancer is sneaky, and what didn't look like cancer on a PET scan was indeed cancer once tested through pathology. The cancer had spread from my breast to my liver.

My body shifted into survival mode, getting stuck in the shock. *I have five years to live? I'm going to die?* My mind raced ahead as I quickly calculated what our children's ages would be in the next five, seven, and ten years. The numbers involuntarily flashed through my mind like bolts of lightning alongside images of what my children would look like as they grew—graduations, first days of school, lost teeth, driving tests. I mustered a smile at my son as he bounded off the bus, somehow, I was able to ask about his day as I simultaneously felt my future as his mother slipping through my fingers like fine grains of sand.

I filled bowls with fruit and Goldfish crackers for the kids and did the one thing every medical professional warns against—I googled metastatic breast cancer.

Up until this point in my diagnosis, I had only looked at information that directly correlated to (what we thought) was my stage of cancer. You see, my initial scans only showed my original tumor in my left breast. My lymph nodes were all clear, my right breast was unscathed, and so I was diagnosed with stage 2B triple positive breast cancer. I had my port placed, I cut my long blond highlighted hair short, and I started a schedule: twelve weeks of chemotherapy and a year of immunotherapy. With encouragement from a friend, I sent my images off to the Mayo Clinic for a second opinion. It was the height of COVID, so my appointment with the breast oncologist was over video. My husband and I busied our four children with some screen-time, and the two of us crammed around his laptop in our home office. We listened as she agreed with my diagnosis and treatment plan. Near the end of our call, she mentioned that my MRI showed what she referred to as a "shadow" on my liver, but not to worry because it did not present itself as cancer, and that I may want to have it looked at after my cancer treatments were complete. We were set to proceed as planned. I clung to those words—*not cancer*—as if they were a promise. At the time, I believed them. I wanted to believe them. There was already so much to carry, and this shadow felt like something I could set down, at least for a while. Still, a quiet unease settled in. I smiled, nodded, and moved forward, but underneath it all was a flicker of fear I did not know how to name. I trusted their guidance completely and was moving ahead full steam, determined to do whatever it took to get through treatment.

When the google search results filled my phone screen, I couldn't believe what I was reading. *Metastatic breast cancer* meant stage 4. And while I had little experience with breast cancer, outside of Susan Sarandon's character in *Stepmom* and a cousin who had gone through treatment, I did know what stage 4 meant.

Fifteen years earlier, I had watched my mother die of stomach cancer. She went from diagnosis to death in less than five months. That trauma had carved itself into my memory, and now, it surged to the surface with a vengeance. I knew what it meant to watch someone you love deteriorate in front of you, powerless to stop it. Only this time, I wasn't the one watching—it was happening to me.

Her death had changed me in ways I did not fully understand at the time. It left a wound, yes—but also a question that never stopped echoing: *What do I do with this pain?* I did not have an answer then. But now, facing my own diagnosis, that same question returned, louder and more urgent. And with it came the beginnings of something else—something that had lived quietly inside me for years, waiting.

Somewhere deep inside, though, beneath the fear and disbelief, there was a flicker of something I couldn't yet name. All my life, I had carried this quiet certainty that there was a purpose waiting for me. Yes, meeting Kevin and building a life with our four beautiful children has been—and will always be—my greatest joy. But even before that, there had always been something more. A feeling I couldn't quite define, one that tugged at me no matter how fulfilled I appeared on the outside. It wasn't that I longed for a different life, but that I longed to *achieve* something more. That drive to pursue, to accomplish, to rise—it had always lived in me, even as a young girl. Maybe it was my way of outrunning grief, of proving I was still whole despite the loss. Maybe it was my need to fill the silence her absence left behind.

As a young adult, I had channeled that yearning into scholarship pageants. I loved everything about competing: searching for the perfect song to showcase my voice, the elegance of beaded gowns and heels, and the adrenaline of stepping into the spotlight with a smile that could light up a stage. My dream was to become Miss America one day. I believed that would be my purpose, or at least the path to it, until I married and started a family. I trained tirelessly, especially for the interview portion, mastering the art of shaping my thoughts into poised, compelling answers for strangers seated behind tables or scattered throughout auditoriums. I poured years of my life into that dream. So when I was named a runner-up, twice, I was devastated. I tried to appreciate the growth, the experiences, the lessons, but in my heart, I was still left asking: *What was all the work for?* I thought that was my purpose. *Now what?*

It would take years—and a diagnosis of my own—before I began to understand that maybe none of it had been wasted. My mother's death had shattered me, but it also planted something inside me, a fierce need to make meaning out of pain. I never wanted her life, or her death, to feel like a closed door. Somewhere deep within, I carried the quiet promise that if I was ever given the chance, I would turn that heartbreak into something good. That her suffering would not be in vain.

What I once thought was the end of a dream—losing the crown, stepping away from the stage—was actually preparation. Every moment spent finding my voice, standing tall, and speaking with conviction had been shaping me for something I could not yet see. My purpose had always been there, waiting. It just did not look the way I expected.

This realization—that there could be a purpose buried somewhere within my pain—did not come easily. It wasn't a graceful epiphany or some peaceful surrender. It was brutal. Humbling. It came with tears, with anger, with long nights staring at the ceiling, asking *why me?* I didn't want to grow through this. I didn't want this to shape me or teach me anything. I wanted my old life back. I wanted the promises I had made to my children to remain true. I wanted *out*.

But eventually, I understood that if I was going to survive this—not just physically, but emotionally—I had to make a choice. I had to find meaning, not because the pain demanded it, but because *I* did. I know not everyone feels that way, and I respect that deeply. Grief, illness, and trauma do not owe us anything—not perspective, not wisdom, not transformation. But for me, choosing purpose was the only way I could keep the pain from being the final word. It wasn't easy. It was a daily act of courage to believe that something good could still live here. There were moments when that belief felt completely out of reach—when the shattered feeling was so complete, I couldn't imagine putting the pieces back together. But still, somehow, I reached for one.

One day, deep in the haze of chemotherapy, when the weight of it all felt unbearable, I needed to be alone—away from the brave face I wore for my children, away from the noise of well-meaning encouragement, away from the exhaustion of simply surviving. I escaped to the shower, hoping the hot water might wash some of the anguish from my skin, even just for a moment. But as the steam curled around me and the water poured over my bald head, everything I had been holding back—every unspoken fear, every swallowed scream—came rushing out.

I pounded my fists against the cold tile wall, overcome with rage, sadness, and disbelief. My sobs were guttural, primal—hot tears mingling with the spray as I cried out to God, "Why is this happening?" My mind scrambled, desperate to make sense of what felt senseless. *How could this be real? How could this happen to me?* There was no clarity in that moment—only the rawness of grief and the ache of a life interrupted.

And yet, even in the breath that followed those broken cries, something stirred. Not peace—not yet—but the faintest glimmer of what might one day become it. It wasn't comfort, but it was something close to recognition. I had already, despite everything, experienced flashes of grace, tiny moments of connection, the kind of unexpected purpose that sneaks in through the cracks of devastation. The truth is, even when I felt crushed beneath the weight of it all, some part of me still hoped. Not because it was easy, but because hope was the only thing left I hadn't tried to let go of.

So, in the many nights following my stage 4 diagnosis, I would lie awake in the dark next to my husband in the glow of my iPhone as I searched for that hope and maybe even some answers to my metastatic questions. I was unable to even formulate my questions early on in my diagnosis. *What exactly am I looking for?* I would wonder. What popped up was not good news: metastatic breast cancer ten-year survival rates were at 13 percent. Metastatic breast cancer five-year survival rates were at 22 percent. Metastatic breast cancer two-year survival rates were at 56 percent. I felt the panic rise as I laid next to my sleeping husband. How long had the cancer been in my body before we found it? Had I already burned through some of those years without knowing? I then decided I should dig my way out of the survival rate rabbit hole, as it only made me feel panicked. I swiped closed the search engine results and opened up Instagram, instead, tapping on the tiny magnifying glass. My thumbs spelled out "breast cancer," and I was greeted with a tidal wave of pink tutus, fuchsia boxing gloves and matching ribbons, survivor sashes, bald heads, and smiles, smiles, smiles. *How are they all smiling?* I wondered as I continued to scroll. *Ugh.* I began sifting through profiles of women who listed "survivor" in their profile bios, but there were just so many women. Screen after screen of women staring back at me, some very obviously were still in the trenches of their cancer, some were sporting their "chemo curls" and were a little way out from their treatment, and then there were others who did not look at all like what I thought they would: young. I scrolled through endless profiles, narrowing my search to HER2, MBC, and triple positive. One woman caught my attention—she was stunning, vibrant, and looked like she had just stepped off the set of a swimsuit shoot. "Living Well w/ Metastatic Breast Cancer," her bio read. "Inspiring you to do what you dream." I wanted—needed—to know if she had my subtype. *Wow. Maybe if she did, I could be like her—I could outlive the statistics.* I felt the first real glimmer of hope. I followed her for hours that night, clicking through her posts, watching her stories, absorbing every word she shared. Her existence didn't erase the statistics, but it challenged them—and that gave me something to hold onto. A thread. A spark. Maybe I could be an outlier too. Maybe I wasn't completely powerless. But as the days unfolded, reality kept sneaking back in.

* * *

After my metastatic diagnosis, it felt like the sky was always falling. I would be outside playing with my kids, my stomach in knots, wondering how we got to this place of uncertainty—specialty pharmacy calls, my very own oncologist, and my mortality constantly being shoved in my face. I could grasp a hold of nothing. The constant worry of what, if, and when, the heaviness of carrying it all, felt like it was about to break me. I needed something to help me feel okay. I tried to figure my way out of this as if I were in an escape room, but the clues were clinical trials, and the key was a cure that only existed for the participants who had arrived earlier in the day.

My reality was that I would not be getting out of the escape room; I would need to be okay with being locked in and settle into how to adjust. I used to take pride in the fact that I did not rely on a single pill for anything. No multivitamins, no calcium supplements, not even acetaminophen unless I had a splitting headache. I envisioned myself aging naturally, without what I once saw as artificial crutches. I believed that with enough determination—and maybe a little magnesium before bed—I could manage whatever came my way. I could exercise more, meditate, do yoga, breathe through it. I thought all I needed was willpower and grit. I thought I could power through this diagnosis with little more than a tightened ponytail and my medical team behind me.

But cancer, as it turns out, is not something you power through. It stripped away the illusion that strength meant doing it alone. I had spent so long trying to be the smiling, waving version of myself—the one who could balance it all, even on the days that left me hollow. I was rushing home from chemotherapy to pick up my youngest kids from school, pretending nothing had changed. I was freezing the meals that friends dropped off, saving them for when things got "really hard," as if that moment had not already arrived.

Eventually, I had to admit the truth: I was afraid. Not just of the cancer, but of what it meant to let others see me struggle. I asked my doctor for help with the relentless anxiety that kept me up at night. I stopped freezing the lasagnas friends dropped off—I cooked them. I let the kindness in. And in doing so, I learned that real strength is not found in pretending everything is fine—it is found in saying yes to help, to rest, to relief, and to love, in all the forms it shows up.

Once I began taking a prescription for anxiety, I realized that my need for control might be greater than I had ever acknowledged. Like many people, I feel better when life feels manageable, predictable even. Being diagnosed with cancer made that crystal clear. I had always believed I liked spontaneity, that I could go with the flow, but in reality, I was deeply uncomfortable with uncertainty. The diagnosis made me incredibly anxious. It felt like I was suddenly dropped into the middle of the ocean—no life raft, no break from the endless treading. Just me, alone, fighting against waves I couldn't control. I had spent years carefully crafting a streamlined life. I was on track to live well and grow old—no handful of pills, no walker waiting in the wings.

* * *

It wasn't easy for me to admit, but deep down, I had always believed that if I did everything "right"—ate well, exercised, stayed on top of my health—I could somehow steer my life in the direction I wanted. Just like during all those pageants I participated in, I believed that if I smiled and answered the questions correctly, I'd win. But as it turns out, life doesn't always work that way. Some things are within our control—the small, seemingly inconsequential choices, like whether to wear a blue or green shirt or whether to schedule a teeth cleaning in the morning or afternoon. But the big things? The ones that truly shape our lives? Those are often completely out of our hands.

About six months into my diagnosis, I started to feel a new anxiousness. Not one of worry necessarily, but one that was brought on by all I was learning from living with incurable cancer. I realized I needed to do more—something that would ground me, something to help me channel the fear, the anger, the deep, gnawing feeling that my life had been ripped out from under me. Late at night, when sleep refused to come (thanks to the joys of medically induced menopause at thirty-eight), I scoured every online resource I could find about metastatic breast cancer. It wasn't enough to just take the treatments and hope for the best—I needed to understand what was happening to my body when I took them. I wanted to know what my doctors were talking about. I needed to arm myself with knowledge, so I could adequately prepare for whatever was coming. Because if I couldn't control the disease itself, maybe, just maybe, I could control how I faced it.

I needed to understand the biology of the disease, the patterns of progression, and the treatments that offered even a sliver of hope. I needed to learn what things were within my control—my attitude, my advocacy, my voice—and what wasn't, like how the cancer might spread or how long I'd have to raise my children. I sought out every resource: research articles, patient forums, support groups, and expert panels. I didn't do this in response to an overwhelming despair, but to equip myself to live *well*. To live with intention, with clarity, and yes—with purpose. Because if this disease was going to be part of my story, I wanted to write the rest of it on my own terms. I decided that if I couldn't control the disease itself, maybe, just maybe, I could control how I faced it.

The more I learned, the more I realized just how much I hadn't known about breast cancer before my diagnosis. I mean, why would I? What I thought I knew about breast cancer—the pink ribbons, the 5Ks, the triumphant survivors crossing finish lines surrounded by cheering friends and family—wasn't the full picture. The media had fed me two versions of this disease: the smiling, pink-clad warriors celebrating survivorship, and the frail, bald, hospital-bound mother in blockbuster movies, clinging to life in a dimly lit room. Neither of those images looked like me. I wasn't on a neatly packaged journey with a finish line and a feel-good victory within my focus. I was existing in something much messier, something that didn't fit into the awareness campaigns or the scripted Hollywood portrayals.

What unsettled me even more was the realization that I had spent my whole life believing breast cancer was something that happened to other people. In 2016, after my mother died from an unrelated cancer, I took genetic tests that screened for over 100 known gene mutations. My results were clear. I had no mutations or genetic red flags. That, I thought, meant I was in the clear. I believed breast cancer was something that happened to women with a family history—something passed down like an heirloom, unavoidable if it was in your bloodline and nonexistent if it wasn't. I had trusted that science could tell me if I was at risk. And yet, here I was. Thirty-eight years old; a runner, healthy eater with no genetic predisposition. And here I was, holding a stage 4 breast cancer diagnosis. How was that possible?

As I dug deeper, I uncovered facts that shattered every assumption I'd had about who gets this disease, and the hows and whys. I learned that metastatic breast cancer—the only form of breast cancer that kills—is responsible for 97–99 percent of breast cancer deaths. Yet, it receives only 3–5 percent of breast cancer research funding. I learned that despite all the conversations I'd heard about genetic mutations being a leading cause, our genes only account for 8–10 percent of breast cancer cases.

Why, then, had I been led to believe that genetic testing was the key to prevention? Why weren't women being told that they could develop breast cancer in their twenties, even without a family history? Why weren't we educated about risk factors beyond genetics?

I thought back to my annual gynecology exams, where I was told I had dense breast tissue. At the time, I thought it was a benign, almost cosmetic observation—maybe even a good thing. Perkier longer, right? What I didn't know—what nearly every woman I've spoken with since didn't know—was that dense breast tissue can mask tumors on mammograms and is, itself, a risk factor for breast cancer. How was I, an educated woman who took charge of my health, so uninformed about something that was quite literally killing me? And if I was unaware, that probably meant most women were.

I knew that as long as I was alive, I had to change that.

I needed an outlet for the flood of information I was gathering. I needed somewhere to put all of this frustration, all of this urgency, all of this raw determination to do something to change things. While I wouldn't call cancer a "gift" (and please, for the love of all things holy, don't tell me that "everything happens for a reason"), I do believe that I can make something purposeful out of this pain because I believe that God does not want harm for me.

After many sleepless nights and page after page of research and information making its way into my inbox, I decided that this terrible, devastating diagnosis would not be wasted. I couldn't let it mean nothing. I've always been comfortable speaking in front of a crowd, so I decided I would tell my story to anyone who would listen. I would show them what breast cancer really looks like—not just the pink ribbons and finish lines, but the burns from radiation, the lifelong treatments women have to endure, the paradox of living with an incurable disease while looking "fine" on the outside. I would shine a light on the way money is funneled into breast cancer campaigns that make people feel good but do little to actually save lives.

I was fueled by anger—anger that the research dollars were out there, but they weren't being directed toward what actually mattered. That the narrative about breast cancer was so sanitized, so misleading, that it left people like me blindsided.

So, I took that anger into my hands in order to keep it from festering in my heart, and I did something with it.

Nearly immediately after my de novo diagnosis in 2020 (meaning from the beginning because my metastasis was not a recurrence), the answer became painfully clear, and I knew, God and science willing, I would not sit idle. How did I go thirty-eight years as a woman who prided herself on being healthy and active know so little about breast cancer? I had switched my focus from pageant queen to semi-crunchy mom who enjoyed homemade kale chips and was vigilant about my well-checks. Other women needed to know what I had learned. I was equipped to deliver my message; all the years I had spent honing my interview skills had been for something—to speak, to educate, to advocate.

Let me be clear—this understanding did not arrive gently. At first, I wrestled with it, fists clenched around the life I thought I was promised. The idea that purpose could rise from something so cruel felt insulting. I paced through denial like a house I refused to leave, slamming doors behind me, unwilling to look at what stood outside. But grief, persistent as breath, kept following me room to room. And somewhere along the way, I stopped fighting long enough to see it: even here, in this broken place, something good could grow. That realization demanded action. If something good could grow, I had to be the one to plant it. I couldn't sit with this knowledge—this ache—and do nothing. I was carrying too much: the weight of my own diagnosis, the faces of friends who were slipping away, the broken promises hidden in pink ribbons. I didn't have a roadmap, just a feeling—an urgency that wouldn't let me rest.

That's where *vraniCURE* began. Not as a perfectly crafted plan, but as a response to heartbreak. A way to take all the pain, the unanswered questions, and the unbearable losses and turn them into something that might help someone else breathe a little easier. I needed something to hold onto—something bigger than my fear, more lasting than my diagnosis. I needed hope, not just for me, but for all of us still here, still fighting.

vraniCURE, a nonprofit that raises funds for metastatic breast cancer research, educates and brings awareness to the disease, and supports the women living with it, because it felt absolutely ludicrous to be in the position I was in and do nothing about it. I was watching my friends die while I was still waking up to run a 5K most mornings. Maybe that's survivor's guilt, or maybe that is how we make peace with our guilt, by turning it into purpose. But it also came from heartbreak—deep, gut-wrenching heartbreak that so many of us were diagnosed too late, misled by pinkwashed campaigns, or told we were "lucky" because we "caught it early," only to find ourselves in stage 4 months or years later. That heartbreak lit a fire in me. I could not stay silent. I began researching how to start a nonprofit from scratch— reading, making calls, asking questions late into the night. I reached out to trusted friends and professionals who shared my urgency and vision, and together, we formed a board of directors. Each of them brought something different to the table—legal insight, business strategy, nonprofit experience, or just a fierce love for someone affected by this disease. It was overwhelming at times—the paperwork, the regulations, the fear that I might be in over my head—but something in me knew I had to keep going. vraniCURE was born not just out of hope, but out of defiance. It was my way of saying: we deserve better. And I was going to do everything in my power to make that happen.

And then there were the women—Lindsey, Jodi, Heather, and Kelsey—who became part of my life because we shared the same diagnosis. These women's lives were full of light and strength and hope, and they should still be here. Losing them shattered something in me, but it also sharpened my resolve. I carry their names in my heart everywhere I go; their stories, legacies, unfinished lives—they are woven into the fabric of vraniCURE. They are the reason I keep speaking, keep fighting, keep showing up. And alongside them are the countless women still living with this disease, who carry its invisible weight with strength and grace. I do this for them too.

Founding vraniCURE gave me something to hold onto; a way to take all of this pain and turn it into purpose. I now have a mission that, no matter what happens to me, will carry their names—and mine— forward into something that matters.

* * *

The sun is making its way back higher in the sky after a long, unforgiving Minnesota winter. The light is sharper now, reflecting off patches of melting snow, forcing me to reach for my sunglasses as I make my way home from the dog park. The air still holds a lingering crispness, but there's warmth too—the kind that hints at spring's slow but certain arrival. I can't help but to feel the symbolism in my diagnosis and the arrival of a new spring.

As I walk, I catch a glimpse of my reflection in a car window. I notice my collared shirt is unbuttoned just enough for my eyes to land on my nearly invisible port scar on my chest. It catches my attention, as it always does. I shift my gaze downward as I recall all the mornings I have found myself running my fingers along the faint, white lines scattered across my chest and back. These scars—silent markers of unimaginable struggles overcome and survived—have softened with time, but they still hold my attention when I stand in front of a mirror. My body, once unfamiliar and foreign after surgeries and treatments, now nearly feels like mine again.

My hair, longer now, is pulled into a snug ponytail that sways back and forth over my shoulder as I turn to smile at my rescue pup trotting beside me. He looks up with the kind of adoration only a dog can give, and I can't help but laugh. I am happy. Genuinely, unequivocally happy. Life is good.

And yet, even in this moment of peace, I realize the past lingers—because it's not truly past. Breast cancer is now part of my every day. Treatment isn't a chapter I can close; it's woven into the rest of my life. The memory of that phone call—the one that split my world into a before and after—still replays more often than I'd like to admit.

But even so, I am here. I am living. And I'm learning that joy and pain can exist side by side: my oncologist's voice, steady but heavy, delivering the words that would change everything; the way the world seemed to shrink in an instant, the air leaving my lungs as I struggled to process what was being said; the way time seemed both excruciatingly slow and terrifyingly fast all at once.

Now, five years beyond that day, I often think about the woman I was when I answered that call. I wish I could go back and hold her hand. I would tell her to take a deep breath. That there's still a road ahead—bumpy, unpredictable, sometimes unbearably hard—but that we are *still on it*. Not only are we surviving, but we are *thriving*. There will be more tears than she can imagine, but also more laughter, more love, more joy, and more adventure than she ever thought possible in those early, dark days.

I'd tell her that, yes, she will still get up before the sky is awake to run and catch a beautiful sunrise. That her legs will feel different and not what they once were, but still strong, her lungs full of air, her body moving not just for the sake of survival but because it *wants* to. And that when she does this, she will feel a new appreciation for it.

I'd tell her that there will be unexpected gifts along the way. Not the kind tied with ribbons, but the quiet, sacred kind that reveal themselves slowly—sometimes in the middle of grief, sometimes in the stillness that follows. Yes, I did say rescue pup. But I won't ruin the surprise just yet—I'll let her discover how he finds us. It involves a hospital stay that stretches too long and a stuffed, fluffy puppy from a dear friend. He'll become more than a pet—he'll become comfort, companionship, and joy in a time that feels anything but joyful.

And he's just the beginning. There will be other gifts, just as unexpected. A deeper clarity about what matters. A tenderness for herself she never thought she'd learn. Relationships that deepen, or arrive unlooked for, and offer the kind of presence that doesn't flinch at suffering. Cancer will take much—but it will also give her the eyes to see beauty she once overlooked, the courage to speak truths she used to silence, and the strength to hold both joy and sorrow without needing to resolve either.

And I'd tell her, above all else, that she is not alone. That she never has been, and she never will be. Even in the moments that feel the most isolating—the scans, the side effects, the nights when fear creeps in—there is a sisterhood quietly holding her up. This community of women may be the club no one ever wanted to join, but it's filled with the fiercest, most generous hearts. The ones who understand without explanation. The ones who show up when the world grows quiet. The ones who teach you how to carry both grief and gratitude without apology.

It turns out, there are gifts waiting in the ruins—gifts I never would've chosen, but ones that have changed me in ways I now treasure. Cancer stripped my life bare, but in doing so, it revealed what was solid beneath the surface. It gave me the eyes to notice the little things—like the way my rescue pup watches me with unwavering trust, or how the sun feels warmer after a round of chemo. It gave me the courage to say what matters, to love without holding back, to live even with the knowledge that the past will never fully be in the past.

My life's work now looks nothing like what I once imagined. But it is work that matters. Work rooted in pain, yes—but also in hope, in community, in something sacred. I am proud to speak up, to fight for more time, more research, more dignity for every woman walking this path. I carry their stories with mine. I honor them as I go.

It is not the life I expected. But it is full of meaning. It is full of connection. And I am lucky—so incredibly lucky—to still be here, doing the work, telling the truth, and choosing joy wherever I can find it.

And when I look at how far I've come, I know this: The story isn't over yet—and as long as I'm here, I'll keep living it with open hands and an open heart.

AUTHOR BIO

Jacquelyn Vranicar is a wife, mother of four, and founder of vrani-CURE, a nonprofit dedicated to funding metastatic breast cancer research, raising awareness, and supporting those living with the disease. Diagnosed de novo metastatic at thirty-eight, she turned a devastating diagnosis into a mission to drive change. Her nonprofit has funded lifesaving research across the country, including work with world-renowned scientists at the University of Minnesota, and provides care packages for women undergoing breast cancer surgery and treatment.

She lives in Minnesota with her family and their rescue dog. Outside of her nonprofit work, she enjoys being a full-time chauffeur for her children, traveling, spending time at the lake, and taking walks with her dog. An avid reader and passionate public speaker, she finds purpose in her pain and is committed to doing as much as she can for metastatic breast cancer for as long as she can.

DEBORAH HUTCHISON

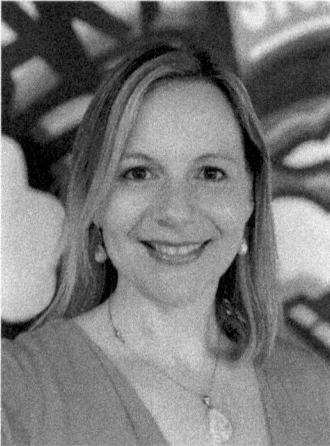

Tears gently rolling down my cheeks, Jason and I held hands as the night closed in around us, our ears tuned to the steady rhythm of the heart monitor. Beep. Beep. Beep. How could this beautiful new life be growing in my belly while at the same time cancer cells are multiplying in my chest? How could new life and possible death exist so closely together? Exhausted, I closed my eyes, as for now all I could do was wait, lie still, surrender to the brokenness, and . . . breathe.

JUST BREATHE

Beep, beep, beep . . . It's all so surreal . . . beep, beep, beep . . . As I float in and out of consciousness, the rhythmic sound of the cardiac monitor keeps bringing me back as a strong, steady reminder that there is still life. Maybe for me, but definitely for her.

I feel a soft and familiar touch—Jason's fingers gently intertwined with mine. I long for the comfort of our own bed, the feeling of being safely tucked under the comforter we have shared since law school. Instead, I am in a hospital bed, covered only by a thin, starchy white sheet, and an equally thin blanket that has long lost its warmth. It is so well intended, that gesture, when you first arrive at the hospital, the nurse pulling a blanket from the warmer and draping it over you like a silent promise of relief: "You're safe now." But the warmth dissipates quickly, and the softness is replaced by another layer of scratchy starch accompanied by the sterile smell of hand sanitizer. I squeeze Jason's hand tighter. None of that matters. What matters is that we are still here. All three of us. Still holding on. It's been six weeks since that dreadful day in August when I thought I would lose her to preterm labor just as I had lost him almost two years earlier. After losing our son, I didn't know if I would ever hold a child of my own. So to be here now, listening to her steady heartbeat is nothing short of a miracle.

Even as I just learned that my body had betrayed me again—this time with breast cancer—her tiny kicks reminded me: it still carries life. I rest my hand on my belly, hoping the warmth of my touch will somehow reassure her that I am here. I close my eyes and try to ground myself in every roll and movement, each one a welcome signal as if she is responding to me—*I am still here, Mama.* In that quiet exchange, I made her a promise: *I will fight for you, my love. With all that I have and all that I am, I will fight.*

That promise to fight echoes through every breath I take but it didn't start here. It began with him—Alexander. Our firstborn. Our son.

Eclipse

Alexander was born too soon. We were living in Kigali then—Rwanda's capital in the "Land of a Thousand Hills." Life felt full and purposeful. We were part of a close-knit expat community, doing work that mattered, and sharing quiet evenings hand-in-hand under the expansive African sky. When we found out I was pregnant, we were over the moon. Ready to share our adventures, our love, our lives with a child. A dream that began to fray that Sunday evening when I felt a dull ache grow in my lower back. Slow at first, ignorable—or so I thought. I was only twenty-five weeks along. I tried to will it away, convincing myself it was Braxton-Hicks contractions, a rehearsal for something far in the future. But with every hour the ache deepened and I just knew something was wrong.

The next morning, I was first in line at the small private hospital tucked into the Kigali suburbs. My heart was racing as the obstetrician spread the gel over my belly in preparation for an ultrasound. She looked up at me with reassuring eyes from under her patterned head scarf as if to let me know it would be okay. I badly wanted to believe she was right. Soon after, we heard our son's heart beat—loud, steady, and strong. It was a deep contrast to how I was feeling, gripped by fear as the aching intensely creeped forward around my pelvis. Still trying to hold on to hope, I repeated in my head, *He's fine, I'm fine, it will all be fine*, like a mantra I could not quite believe. Then came the news—my cervix was failing, my body was giving way too soon. *I was failing.*

I desperately clung to the illusion that maybe if I did everything just right, I could somehow hold off the inevitable? Maybe if I just steadied my breathing, laid on my left side, had some more water, maybe my heart wouldn't shatter. But my rebelling body didn't listen—minute by minute, I was losing greater control. The contractions surged. Our son was coming, ready or not. And as my pregnancy unraveled so did my sense of self-worth. *I was failing.*

As I went into full labor, one nurse took her position on my right side holding up one leg, while another moved to my left. There were no stirrups, no epidurals, no time to prepare, to process, to grieve what was happening. Jason held my hand as I squeezed tightly, both our eyes filled with fear and pain. "This is not how this is supposed to go!" I sobbed, surrounded by a makeshift birthing team of my colleague, the US embassy nurse, and a top Harvard-trained neonatologist who happened to be in Rwanda on a short training mission. My community had shown up. They did everything they could, but I couldn't do the one thing *I* was supposed to do—protect my son. Control my body. Keep him safe. *I had failed.*

After just a few desperate pushes, he was born. Our son. Our angel, born too soon. For a few long minutes, his warm, tiny body was laid on my chest—skin to skin—swaddled with nothing but my everlasting, unconditional love. Through my tears, I kissed his forehead, and whispered, "I love you so much. Just breathe, my love."

I must have passed out, because the next time I opened my eyes it was to the sharp smell of antiseptic and the cold sting of reality. *Where is all this blood coming from?* A nurse was mopping the floor around and beneath me and then I realized the blood was mine—I was hemorrhaging. But there was no time for recovery, I needed to rally. A small medical plane had been commissioned for an emergency evacuation. This was Alexander's only chance to survive. I needed to pull myself together and appear stable enough to fly. I forced myself to focus. *I can do this. I have to do this. I can take back control.* Without a second thought, I signed consent to prioritize his life over mine. There wouldn't be enough staff nor equipment on board to care for us both. I walked as steadily as I could out of the hospital, onto the tarmac. Each step, an act of sheer determination. Once on board, covered by a warm blanket, I finally exhaled. While I could not hold him, for almost four hours on that flight to Johannesburg, I sat beside him. And in that narrow, humming plane, I had the gift of time with my son. The longest stretch we ever shared.

Beep, beep, beep ... the next day, I woke up ... alone. Now in a state-of-the-art facility, it was clear I had survived. Too weak to walk, a nurse wheeled me to the NICU. As we rolled through the maternity ward, I hoped that maybe I, too, would get to hold my baby again. Then, I saw him—wires and tubes draped over, into and out of his tiny body; his preemie diaper swallowing him whole. So small. So brave. So deeply loved.

I pressed my hand to the glass of the incubator, whispering through my tears, "Mommy is here, my love." *Beep, beep, beep* ... the monitor told me he was still fighting. But the nurse suddenly wheeled me to the side of the room and drew the blue curtains, separating my boy from me. *Beep, beep . . . beep . . . . beep . . . .* The rhythm faltered. *Beep . . . . beep . . . .* My heart pounded in my chest as I sifted through the layers of starchy fabric on my lap, and absently wondered where my warm blanket was. Then she slowly opened the curtain again, stepped forward and placed our baby boy in my arms. He was still. No more beeps. No more fight. No more breath. I kissed his cold cheeks and held his lifeless body close against mine. *Breathe, Alexander, please . . . just breathe,* I begged him.

Time stood still in that moment, never to be forgotten. The grief never left, it simply reshaped itself with time. The guilt underneath, grounded in failure, bitterly lingered. I would never fail like that again—not as a woman, a wife, or a mother.

Failure

Failure has always terrified me. Not only the type of failure when you get something wrong, but a deeper fear of not being good enough. Not smart enough. Not pretty enough. Not accomplished enough. Not worthy and lovable enough. It showed up everywhere—in school, where I chased the perfect grades; with my friends, where I tried desperately to fit in; at work, where achievement became my identity.

As I search for the roots of my relentless fear of failure, I wonder if maybe it is generational—woven into my story even before it began. Maybe it began with my grandparents, whose dreams were reduced to rubble during World War II. Maybe with my parents, who worked so hard to build a better life for us, always fighting their way up. Maybe it is from the nuns in Catholic school, where sin seemed a given and worthiness must be earned. Maybe it was the law school professor, who told us on our first day, "Look to your left. Look to your right. Most of you won't make it."

Some days the fear could be paralyzing. One stray worry could throw me into a downward spiral of what-ifs. I fought back my fears not by processing but by pushing through the only way I knew how: work harder, be better, survive. That mindset had carried me for so long, and so far, it had served me well. It had built the foundation for my self-worth. I had earned graduate degrees on three continents, climbed the corporate ladder, and successfully pivoted to pursue my passion in international development. If you work hard enough and push through, the outcome will follow. Maybe not perfectly, but close enough. "Shoot for the moon," my favorite coffee mug used to say, "Even if you miss, you'll land among the stars." It didn't say anything about aiming high and plummeting into the darkness instead.

Corona

And now, here I am back in the United States, less than two years after Alexander's sudden arrival and devastating departure. I was given another chance to do it *right*. On the dresser beside me was the chalkboard we used to track each passing day of my bed rest. Six weeks had passed since preterm labor had once again tried to steal away our baby. Six weeks of holding my breath. But now, I am thirty-four weeks along and I had done everything right—a cervical cerclage to reinforce my "incompetent cervix," weekly progesterone shots, a delirium-inducing magnesium drip, and steroid shots to speed up our girl's lung development, just in case. *This time, I will not fail.*

Just as I started to believe it, the bottom fell out—again. I felt a pressure in my right breast, deep and misplaced. I ran my finger tips over my skin and there it was—a lump. A wave of fear crashed over me, leaving me nauseous and panicked. I tried not to spiral but I knew not to dismiss it. Not even when my regular ob-gyn waved it off as probably just a clogged milk duct—nothing unusual while pregnant. But after everything I had been through, the unimaginable was not theoretical for me. For me it had a name, a face, a touch, a memory.

So I listened to the whispers telling me to not let this go unchecked and scheduled the appointment. And sure enough the ultrasound technician's ghostly face gave it all away. The cold gooey gel turned to ice as she moved it around my chest with the transducer. Up, down, a bit more to the right, pushing in a bit harder in certain spots, and then stopping to click away and get more images. "I'll be right back," she had said with a tight smile. Another lab coat, another set of nitrile gloves moving the transducer around my breast. More images. "This does not look good," the doctor said matter of factly. "We need to do a biopsy to confirm." I rubbed my belly, hoping it might somehow shield my daughter from the fear that was consuming me.

The days and nights between the biopsy and the results were long. As I waited for the diagnosis, I braced for the worst. I tried to distract myself working on my laptop while propped up in bed by the body-sized pregnancy pillow. Then, my phone rang. It was late. *Doctors don't call after hours with good news. Good news can wait until tomorrow.* Sure enough, there it was—the Diagnosis—"You have invasive ductal carcinoma," she said.

Cancer. One dreadful word confirmed my fears and shattered my world. My fragile hope to reclaim motherhood, suddenly thrown into question—again. *What about my baby?* I knew that as long as she was okay, I could find the strength to endure the pain, the fear, the relentless uncertainty. But the possibility of losing her, I could not survive. Not again.

Clutching my belly with one hand and the phone in my other, I called my high-risk ob-gyn. She had helped me temper my anxious mind with the best modern medicine had to offer while allowing my heart to heal as my belly grew. *She will know what to do.* And sure enough, she knew exactly what I needed: a safe space, a warm blanket and . . . a heart monitor. "Go to the hospital, I will meet you there," she ordered.

Beep, beep, beep. Jason's hand is holding mine as I look at the heart monitor strapped around my big pregnant belly. Our daughter's heart beat steady and strong. I pull out my phone and record the sound so it may help me remember that this time, things are different. This time, I will not fail. Our daughter will live, and I will not let this breast cancer diagnosis stop either of us.

She admitted me for the night in the same maternity ward, possibly the same room, where just six weeks ago I had begged my body to hold on and keep our baby safe a little while longer. Opposite the hospital bed, the butterfly decal still declared, "Every day is a gift." Tonight, it has taken on a new meaning. Then, it was a hope-filled promise. Now, a countdown. *How many days do I have left? Will she make it through this? Will I? Will I see my daughter grow up?*

As I tried to stop myself from spiraling, I scanned the room searching for something else to anchor me. My eye caught a poster by the door—it was a public health announcement with a reminder of the critical benefits of breastfeeding, something I would never get to do now. Tears gently rolling down my cheeks, Jason and I held hands as the night closed in around us, our ears tuned to the steady rhythm of the heart monitor. *Beep. Beep. Beep. How could this beautiful new life be growing in my belly while at the same time cancer cells are multiplying in my chest? How could new life and possible death exist so closely together?* Exhausted, I closed my eyes, as for now all I could do was wait, lie still, surrender to the brokenness, and . . . breathe.

Patience is not my strongest suit, and it turns out it isn't our daughter's either. Just five days after my diagnosis, we were back in the hospital. It was time. After the last stitch of my cerclage was removed, my cervix fully lived up to its incompetence. Within a few hours, the familiar rhythm of the contractions, their force and timing grew stronger and closer together. *Here we go again.* My thoughts were heavy, my heart scared knowing it was still five weeks too early for her to join us. But this time nobody was stopping it. No shots, no bedrest, no pleading for one more day. She must be born, simply so I could begin fighting my next battle. She had done her part, my brave little girl, she had grown strong. Now I must do mine. I was terrified but I had to let her come. Not because I had failed at keeping her safe, but because it was the only way I might be able to stay with her.

I declined any pain medicine. Maybe I wanted to feel it all—the pain, the fear, the rush. Maybe I wanted it to feel like last time with Alexander. Maybe I hoped it would somehow bring me closer to him. Maybe I was just plain scared. Maybe, and I am certain I understand this, it will be the last time I feel anything at all. Maybe I just needed to know that I was still alive, and she was too.

And then, as if my body suddenly remembered, pushing through the fear and pain, letting go, she was born. I hold my breath, waiting to hear hers. There it is . . . the sweet sound of her first cry. She did it! She can breathe all by herself! The nurse places her on my chest, and her tiny fingers wrap around mine. Just like her brothers' had. For a moment, the intense pain and agony vanishes, eclipsed by something far greater—an unconditional and overwhelming love for our baby girl Seraphina. A love that transcends every broken piece of me. How remarkably competent was my placenta to have kept her safe from any malignancy. The same body that had failed me before, had done something incredibly right, it had given her life. In this quiet triumph, I allowed myself to just breathe. To let go. Just for a moment before rising again to fight.

As soon as I exhaled, the medical whirlwind began again. We replaced gynecologists with oncologists. Ultrasounds searching for a heartbeat with MRIs, CTs, and PET scans mapping the silent path of deadly cells inside me. Folic acid and magnesium were replaced with chemotherapy and an infusion calendar. Armed with a binder filled with fact sheets and a notebook full of questions, Jason, Seraphina, and I went from doctor's office to doctor's office. We learned an entirely new language—tumor markers, margins, lymph nodes, recurrence risk. We decided on a treatment plan over midnight feedings and scrolled through post-mastectomy reconstruction photos as our baby slept soundly in the surgeon's office. We talked about survival chances, agreed to genetic testing, and tried on wigs. And still, in the quiet spaces in between appointments, we marveled at the gift we had been given. We perfected our swaddling techniques and soaked up our sweet girl's first coos and smiles. My body was preparing for battle, so soon after childbirth, while my heart was overflowing with gratitude for being her mom.

Fight

For my thirty-second birthday, I got a renewed chance at life. *Wouldn't it be poetic to start chemo on my birthday as a symbol of rebirth while staring death in the face?* I tried to convince myself as I looked in the mirror and brushed my fingers through my blond hair. I lingered, knowing I would lose it soon. Maybe that works on TV, but the symbolism of it fell flat the night before Round One. There was no sense of heroism, only trembling. Maybe it was the steroids I was given to prepare my postpartum body for what was to come. More likely it was the fear of not knowing how much I could endure or how much time I had left.

A soft cry saved me from the darkness of my spiraling thoughts—Seraphina was awake again, ready for her next nighttime feeding. I spent the long hours of the night with her, holding her in my arms, rocking her in the chair we had picked out not long ago, when I was still untouched by cancer, when the biggest decision to make had been her crib color: white or driftwood. My heart filled with gratitude for her milky smile, her soft cheeks, her little body bundled tight in her butterfly-covered swaddle. *Just breathe, little one.* I whispered it to her and then to myself, *Just breathe.* I wish I could freeze time, but the first rays of sun had already started to peek through the shades. It was time for chemo. Round One.

Rounds . . . I have always been a fighter. Back in high school, I threw punches to the sound of "Eye of the Tiger" blasting from the speakers. Three rounds, adrenaline soaring with every jab and roundhouse kick, each a sign of strength bringing me closer to victory. But this . . . this was different. There were no Rocky-like vibes. There was no training to prepare me for what was to come. Instead of stepping into the kickboxing ring, I settled into the secluded chemo pod by the window. There were no hand wraps to protect my hands—only a warm hospital blanket to shield me from the cold terrors. Then, a needle, and just the quiet crossing of a line between what life could have been and what it had now become. As I felt the cold liquid from the first of four IV bags slide down my veins, shivers climbed up my spine. My eyes welled up with tears while Jason, ever present, gently held my hand. I didn't resist. I welcomed the loading doses of chemo drugs into my veins, asking them as my allies to seek out all the cancer cells they could devour. I surrendered and closed my eyes. *Happy birthday to me.*

The chemo infusion took all day, a slow drip of poison meant to save me, it left me exhausted. When we finally made it home, there she was—our baby girl sleeping peacefully in her crib. Her chest rising and falling in a steady rhythm. She didn't know the battle I had just started, the silent war that was raging beneath my skin. Nor did she know that she was my salvation. My reason to keep going. She didn't need to. Her being here—breathing—was enough. She was enough. *Just breathe.* I reminded myself and matched my rhythm to hers.

Round Two of chemo also marked the end of my six-week maternity leave. The calendar said it was time to go back to work, but my body was reeling and my mind was still spinning trying to find its center again. *How can I go from a chemo pod to a desk chair, from baby blankets to spreadsheets, from bouts of nausea to break room coffee?* Cancer had already stolen many things from me—my hair, my energy, my hope for a normal maternity leave, one focused on bonding with my baby without fear looming in every quiet moment. But I refused to let it take away my professional purpose too, my drive of doing good in the world. So I drove to work, suppressed my nausea, adjusted my wig in the rearview mirror, and stepped into my role. I spent my days guiding strategy, coaching teams, and increasing program efficiency—so that people I would never meet would one day have access to quality health care, the kind that saves lives. It was more than a job—it was a lifeline, for them and for me. It gave me a sense of control and normalcy over at least one part of my life, and even on my weakest days, it reminded me I still had something meaningful to offer to the world as a modern professional woman, juggling career and motherhood.

I felt accomplished as I put in a full day of work and held my baby at night. *Yes,* I told myself, *I am doing this!* I was striving and surviving. Until I wasn't. Even strength has limits, and I was about to reach mine as I entered Round Three, my knock-out round.

There were no warning signs, and I had no defense. Just the painful truth: my body could no longer bear the weight of the accumulating medicine meant to save it. The chemo flooded my lungs with fluid and drowned the rhythm of my heart. There was no referee to pause the fight, no bell to ring for reprieve, no smelling salts to bring me back to consciousness. I was rushed to the nearest ER, where two nurses frantically tried to find a vein that had not yet collapsed from the chemo. I faded in and out of consciousness while people walked in and out of the room—another test, more drugs, more questions. An oxygen mask strapped on tight. *Beep, beep . . . beep.* The not-so-rhythmic blips of the heart monitor reminded me that I was still there. In the blur, I teetered between life and death. On one side the mother and professional I had fought so hard to become, and on the other my body, betraying me, again, surrendering to a blitzkrieg of a war I never asked to fight.

But I didn't have the luxury of choice. I had to find a way to keep going, not just for me, but most importantly for them. For the little girl, whose future I longed to see unfold. For the little boy, who fought so bravely for his short time in this world. For the loving man, who was always there, as my rock, my pillow, my strength when I had none left.

As the doctors brought me back from the edge—defeated but alive—I knew I desperately needed a new path. For months, I had been fighting with all my might just to survive. Working by day, mothering by night. I followed every medical directive, and even the nonmedical ones—drinking ginger tea to ease the nausea, boiling herbal soups in our kitchen to strengthen my immunity, and pouring my thoughts into my diary in the quiet of the night. I had been doing what I thought was expected of me—staying strong, taking the punches, and getting up, round after round. But lying there, oxygen mask strapped to my face, I wondered: *How long can I keep doing this? When is it enough? When do I get to just breathe, and simply be enough?*

By the time Round Four arrived, I was patched up just enough to return to the chemo ward, physically at least. Inside, I was unraveling.

As the chemo nurse searched my arms for a viable vein, our nurse navigator came over—she was always a calm presence in the storm of my chemo days. "How are you doing, Deborah?" she asked thoughtfully. She already knew the answer by just looking at me—I wasn't just pale, bald, battered, and bruised. I was completely broken. And right there, in a room full of people fighting for their lives, I cracked. I started sobbing uncontrollably. Embarrassed by my obvious lack of control, I began apologizing for the mess I had become. "Stop apologizing," she gently said. "You are going through so much." The softness in her eyes reminded me that she had walked this road too.

"But what about staying strong?" I started, my voice trembling, "Thinking positive? Doesn't that help? Isn't that how we survive this?" *Isn't that what we are told? The warriors wear pink, smile through the struggle, and turn trauma into inspiration.* My thoughts were swirling, genuinely afraid that if I let go of the fight—even for a moment—I would fail and lose the battle. Terrified that if I let the darkness in—even just to process it—it would stay. Her eyes met mine with a calm kindness. I searched for judgment, but there was none. "No," she said gently, "there are no studies that say you need to be strong and positive all the time to survive cancer." She reached out and held me in a quiet embrace; it was a hug that didn't try to fix anything or cheer me up. She sat next to me and taught me her remedy—*saltwater facials*, she called them. Not the kind you book at the spa but the kind you receive from crying your heart out, from letting it all go, from giving yourself permission to feel—all the feelings—the grief, the fear, the rage. The kind that teaches you that healing doesn't always look like hope and heroism. Sometimes, it looks like breaking. That day, I learned that strength isn't about never breaking, never failing. It is about daring to surrender and still be enough. To fall and still rise.

In the weeks, months, and Rounds ahead, saltwater facials became a staple for me. I liked having mine in the shower—where the water would hold me in warmth and solitude. Letting the warm water run over my bald scalp, down my trembling shoulders, across my sensitive chemo skin, I could finally let go. Unleash the emotions I had been holding in as I tried to keep it together for the outside world. I cried—sometimes softly, sometimes loudly, often desperately. I cried for the pain, for the grief of everything I had lost, and the fear of losing everything I had left. Tears flowing freely, mixing with the shower stream, indistinguishable. As I surrendered, everything blended—salt and freshwater, fear and hope, anger and gratitude, loss and love. The water washed away what I could hold no longer—the guilt of not being enough, the fear of being a burden, and the weight of believing I had failed as a mother, a wife, a woman. In this space, I had the courage to surrender without apologizing and felt accepted, if by no one else than the shower gods, who never judged me, never urged me to just be strong or made me question if I was worthy. They just held me until the water ran cold and my tears ran dry.

Equinox

With every saltwater facial, I gave myself permission to be vulnerable, imperfect, and broken. I wasn't looking for results, or clarity, or even healing—not yet. I was just trying to find *neutral* — a place between panic and performance, between despair and pretending. I didn't need to feel strong or do better. Neutral wasn't about giving in. It was about grounding and courage. It was about allowing myself to be rooted just enough to let go and find the strength to rise again. Not to fight but to just breathe.

Neutral didn't change the path ahead—the double mastectomy and then a total hysterectomy that left me with more losses to grieve and the battle scars to remind me; the reconstruction that stretched my skin and my patience; the year-long Herceptin infusions that became a routine reminder of cancer in my calendar and my veins; and the decade-long hormone therapy that presses on, year after year, not as a guarantee but as a daily act of hope in pill form laced with side effects. Neutral didn't make any of that easier, but it gave me a place to return to—a way to move *through* the pain, fear, and uncertainty without always fighting *against* them.

As I couldn't always retreat to the sanctity of my shower, I looked for other places where my breath could steady again, where surrender didn't mean defeat but grace, where enough didn't require achievement but just presence. And slowly, I found them, in the little things.

I found it in the stillness of night, journaling under the veil of darkness, giving myself permission to empty the heaviness on paper and process my deepest thoughts. I found it when rocking Seraphina to sleep, matching my breathing to hers, my heart overflowing with unconditional love.

I found it in the words of the Serenity Prayer, memorized by heart and over time reshaped as my own quiet plea to the universe to give me *the strength to keep going, the courage to let go of what does not serve me, and the grace of unconditional love to just breathe.*

Some days, I found it wearing pink—not for the world, but for myself—as a quiet reminder of my own strength. Still here, still strong. On appointment days, I found it holding a piece of rose quartz tucked in my pocket to help ground me in unconditional love. And when the ache of grief crept in, I reached for my tri-colored gold ring—the one my mom gave me to remind me that Jason, Alexander, and I are forever intertwined. A circle of love that no loss can ever break.

Each of these quiet rituals and imperfect efforts helped me exhale a bit deeper and, little by little, the belief that I have to earn my breath and prove my worth in every moment started to soften. I learned that finding neutral is not a weakness. It is wisdom. It is how I create space—space to heal. Space to live in the balance between striving to win and surrendering to be.

Even now, ten years later, I return to that space again and again. Sometimes in the old familiar ways—hot showers, journaling, a rose quartz in my palm. Other times in new ways—a quiet nature walk, a gentle surrender to movement and breath on the yoga mat, or tracing the moon shaped pendant that holds our family's birthstones, their weight close to my heart, remembering I carry them and they carry me.

Healing, I learned, is incremental. Sometimes it roars—like the day chemo ended. Other times, it hums—like when I trace my daughter's cheek with the back of my hand as she sleeps, or whisper Alexander's name as a white butterfly flutters by, letting its wings carry my love to where my arms no longer can.

Healing is fragmented—uneven, unexpected, and unfinished. The mosaic of me is not one of perfection. It is broken. It is built from tiny pieces—some I fought hard to get, some I thought I had lost, and some I am still discovering—all glued together with breath.

There are jagged pieces of pain—a baby blanket never used, goodbye letters written in the middle of the night, a lock of hair cut at the root before shaving my head. Others are slivers of courage—walking into surgery with head high and heart pounding, knitting one more crooked row in that uneven baby hat, stepping outside with post-chemo stubble catching the sun.

Some pieces shimmer with joy—Seraphina's bathtime giggles, her arms around my neck as she hugs me tight. Some radiate with light—bringing home our youngest, Anastasia, who grew in my heart rather than my belly. Others are dipped in love—Jason's steady hands replacing my bandages, his presence anchoring me when I am lost. And then the unexpected bits—chocolate croissants on appointment days, the waiting room friendships, a tribe built in sisterhood.

Healing hasn't erased my grief, my fear, or the failures that still echo. But it has allowed me to let those pieces live alongside the others. I now honor who I am becoming—a mosaic of grief and joy, failure and resilience, tenderness and strength. This stained glass of pain and survival, courage and surrender, motherhood and womanhood, cracks and vibrant color, is my becoming. And in its fractured light, I cannot only breathe, I can be enough.

AUTHOR BIO

Deborah is a mom, a wife, a professional, and a "wounded healer." Born and raised in Belgium, she became a global citizen when she moved to the United States to continue her studies. She met her husband Jason at Vanderbilt Law School, and they have traveled the world together ever since. Their passion for making a difference in the world has brought them to live and work on four continents.

A lifelong learner and an empathic leader, Deborah has dedicated her career to advancing public health and improving lives. Throughout her career, she has worked with communities from the Philippines to Rwanda, from the fields of healthcare consulting and biotech to academia and international development. Whether helping a young boy access life-saving craniofacial surgery, teaching midwives Kangaroo Care, ensuring HIV or malaria medicines reach those in need, or supporting hospital systems to meet regulatory standards, Deborah is passionate about serving others, wherever they are.

At age thirty-one, Deborah was diagnosed with breast cancer while pregnant with her daughter. After the devastating premature loss of their son, Deborah and Jason were overjoyed for another chance at starting a family. When hearing the words "You have invasive ductal carcinoma"—cancer—her world shattered, again. During her cancer journey, she learned that it is okay to not be okay, to surrender to brokenness, and to just breathe.

Today, as a mother of two strong and beautiful daughters, Deborah continues to live her purpose—leading global health efforts, volunteering in her spare time, and walking alongside others as a wounded healer in their own breast cancer journeys.

LIZ GERBER

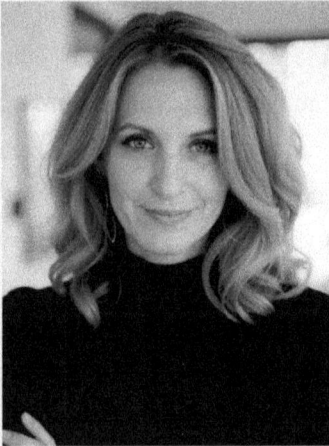

With each subsequent treatment, I would have less good days and more days where I couldn't move, couldn't eat, couldn't walk down the hall without being breathless. The depression and anxiety that had been my lifelong companions took up residence on either side of me, whispering into my ears that this cancer treatment was going to destroy me; that maybe I couldn't make it through. It took all my strength to convince my mind that while it felt like I was dying, in fact, this poison coursing through my veins, was the very thing that would save my life.

STRENGTH REWRITTEN

It's been sixty-six days since I felt a grape-sized lump in the lower part of my breast during a shower. Thirty-two days since I had my breasts smashed between two metal plates followed by an ultrasound where the doctor pointed out the lump had blood flow. He danced around saying the c-word, but that was a sure sign it was malignant. It's been twenty-seven days since I went in for a core needle biopsy, all I can remember is the pain, despite the numbness. And then thirty days since I finally got confirmation over the phone that, yes, I did have cancer.

I have cancer. I had my chemotherapy appointment twelve days ago, on my birthday, no less. I have not lost my hair yet, but it has become dead and lifeless, and I can feel the tingling pain of hair loss in my roots. And now, I am here, staring up at the tiled ceiling of an acupuncture clinic in Chinatown. I wound up here after becoming delirious on painkillers one sleepless night, when the nausea and body pain had become too much to manage. Since high school, I've been drawn to the art of the mind-body connection. Trying something beyond what my oncologist prescribed for me gave me a sense of control over my own body, which has eluded me for exactly thirty days, since I was suddenly someone with cancer.

The doctor is a small Chinese man who had twenty years of practice, he tells me. He quietly listens to me explain why I'm here. "I had my first chemo two weeks ago and since then, I've been sick with nausea and can't eat much. I've also had terrible, burning pain in my bones. And the dry mouth and metallic taste is absolutely awful," I said with increasing frustration. I had put up with feeling abysmal for two weeks and in front of me was another four months of compounding challenges. "I'm hopeful this will provide relief from the relentlessness of feeling so sick," I explain.

He then gently shows me where on my body he wants to place the pins, and explains which meridians and organs it will treat. I lie down on a massage-like table while he puts the needles in place, all along my ankles, and at my temples. One by one, I feel a small pinch as he taps and turns the hypodermic needles. I look around his small office and wonder why the walls only go halfway up. I try to distract myself by eavesdropping on the older woman on the other side of the half-wall speaking Chinese. Of course, I can't understand a word, but I listen anyway. The door chimes as another patient enters. A blast of cold air comes through as the door opens and ushers in frigid March air.

The needles didn't really hurt while he was applying them, but some areas were more sensitive than others, and finally, after many minutes of poking, they were all set. The doctor turned the lights down and instructed me to "just relax." That sounds so easy, but I haven't been relaxed in such a long time. And especially not the last few months. I couldn't really move because of the needles. So, I had no choice but to quietly lay there, listening as the conversations of people I didn't know buzzed around me.

Before I knew what was happening, hot tears forced their way out and streamed down my cheeks, dripping into my ears and pooling in my lifeless hair. There was no throat lump or even a chin quiver to warn me that an emotional outburst was erupting. No one particular thought had made its way into my mind and out through my tears. But it felt as if with each pinprick a release valve had been pressed and my body was so full of grief that when the doctor placed the needles, I must have sprung a leak. And this leak was massive, letting out all that had built up over the last sixty-six days. The diagnosis, the tests, the conversations, the fear, the pain, the unknown, all of it was flowing out of me at the same time.

My body, in its wise and knowing way, was unblocking the trauma that I was holding onto so tightly. I was only at the start of my treatment journey, but that moment allowed me a release and rebalancing from the initial shock. The tears stopped spilling, slowly drying to the sides of my face as the acupuncturist came in to remove the pins and release me back to my reality. I was purged of the initial shock of my diagnosis and now, as I walked to my car in the cold, winter air, I felt an awakening of determination. I would get back into that infusion chair for my second treatment; I would make it out of this diagnosis alive and well.

Chaos is a state of disorder and confusion with no order or pattern. My cancer diagnosis was chaos born out of chaos. The last couple of years, prior to my diagnosis, had been some of the most challenging I could remember. Like most, my 2020 started out with a global pandemic. My husband Matt was teaching high school from the dining room table. I had a three-year-old with no day care (who stopped napping), a full-time job, and involved parents and in-laws most vulnerable to this unknown respiratory disease.

As someone with an anxious brain, the daily mental calculations of keeping myself and my family safe started to wear on my sanity. My mom lived alone and she became very lonely during isolation. My son Nolan was young and we were struggling to keep up with childcare and work. But what if my mom came to help with Nolan and we unknowingly exposed her to COVID? What if I met up with friends and social distanced, but still got Nolan sick? At that time, we still didn't know how the virus impacted young children. The consequences for every decision were just so big. The unknowns in all areas of my life stretched out into oblivion.

That August as COVID life stretched on, my company announced impending January layoffs. I had to wait and work for six months, not knowing if I'd have a job at the end of it. When January finally arrived, I learned my position had been impacted, so I started the grueling process of interviewing. It felt like the uncertainties in my brain were being set up like dominoes. One misstep and the whole line up would fall onto each other until there was nothing left of our lives as we had known them. Then, in late January, what we'd feared for ten months happened. My mother-in-law and father-in-law contracted COVID. One week into testing positive, they both had to be driven by ambulance to the hospital.

At this point in early 2021, vaccines were not yet widely available and families were not allowed to visit in the hospital. Matt spent that first week on the phone with different nurses getting updates on his mom and dad; they were placed in different rooms, not able to speak to each other. Two weeks after testing positive for COVID, my father-in-law Bill passed away after he was put on a ventilator and his kidneys failed. *How could this have happened so fast?* We wondered. Two weeks before, Bill was fine and had talked about registering for his vaccine. We had spent a whole year making calculated decisions on what was safe and not safe, what to trust or not trust. It was devastating. I hadn't lost a parent, so I didn't know how to help my husband work through the grief of his father's death and the anger from the politics of the whole pandemic. We got through that year, but just barely.

Life at that time was heavy. My family was trying to wade through early grief and I was reluctantly job searching, while feeling like a battered ship in the storm. I listened to all the advice on how to "fake it until you make it," but I was swimming in my self-doubt. Every interview was a test of my vulnerability, putting myself in front of a panel of judges whose sole purpose was to score each answer and determine if I was good enough. When the thanks-for-your-time-but-we-found-a-better-fit email hit my inbox, I would spiral into self-pity and it would take me a day or two to recover. Rejection hurts, but after such a painful year filled with loss and tragedy, the consistent messaging that I wasn't enough brought my inner narrative to life, creating a reality that I had worked so hard to keep in the back of my mind.

But, finally a bright spot. I heard the words, "We'd like to offer you a role on the brand team." I had been trying to make a career pivot and now here it was. I felt relief and optimism for the first time in over a year. The next nine months I worked harder than ever, learning a new role and feeling challenged again. In December, I took time off for the holidays so I could finally slow down, take a breath, and reset. "I think this will be the year we can stop treading water and finally look forward," I told my husband. But I think I jinxed it. After sleeping in and taking a late shower, I felt that grape sized lump. My gut told me I was about to face something I couldn't imagine. My world was upside down, again.

Those few weeks after getting my official cancer diagnosis were some of the most consequential weeks of my life. Every test, every outcome, every conversation holds so much weight to what happens next. This is the point where my doctor staged my cancer, identified how aggressive it was, if it had spread to my bones or other parts of my body, and if I would need chemo. *Waiting* is the word that flashes red when I look back at that time.

I was both numb and emotional, bursting into tears thinking about daily events with my son, but then telling coworkers and family my news with an upbeat message that I would get through this. When I said the words, I believed them, until I was alone again with my thoughts. The reemergence of the unknowns, this time with my life at stake, buried me. Throughout all the waiting, I was holding onto a life line that I would not need chemo. In my mind, the hair loss, nausea, and fragility were visual representations of someone battling cancer. I couldn't be that vulnerable and open with my struggles. I was not a strong enough person. But, in life, we don't always get to choose when or how we fight our battles. My test results came back HER2-positive. I would need chemo and it would be the first step in my treatment plan.

When I look back at that time, I saw cancer as the biggest challenge of my entire life. And in many ways, it was. There was something sobering and vulnerable when I realized I was not immune to death. Even if I made it through treatment and became NED (no evidence of disease), cancer is a chronic illness. It could sneak back into my life at any time and catch me off guard again. But I knew what it was like to struggle with chronic disease. I had been silently struggling with another illness since my early twenties; depression and anxiety. I can't sort out which one came first, but my first real experience with it was in college, where it took up residence inside my heart and mind.

Once my treatment plan was determined, my oncologist moved with swift action. I had nine days to prepare myself for my first chemo infusion. During that week and a half, I signed papers informing me of all the side effects of my chemo and immunotherapy regimen. I signed a living will, which brought my unspoken fears of my diagnosis front and center. And then when I had surgery to place my port, the full reality became clear. In less than a week, I would have chemo drugs running directly into my heart and veins.

I was a ball of nerves, fragile, tears pricking my eyes day and night. Matt did all he could that week, but I could tell he was just as shell shocked as I was. His way of coping was to step back and quietly support me from the background. Over that week, the tension built. I was craving someone to take the lead, coordinate doctors appointments, learn about managing side effects, and just help shoulder some of the emotional burden. I see now, my expectations were based on how I would handle the situation if roles were reversed; maybe it was a little unrealistic. Matt was overwhelmed with managing his own emotions and keeping up the daily life chores, as well as communicating with family. But, I was also drained to my soul, and in my mind, I needed someone to carry me over that first, formidable chemo obstacle.

I walked into the cancer center on February 25 at 7 a.m. and checked in for my first chemotherapy and pre-appointment with my oncologist. I gave the receptionist my name and date of birth. She looked up at me and flashed a big wide smile. "Wow, happy birthday!" she announced as if I were checking in for a nice dinner and not a daylong chemo session. "Yeah, thanks," I answered quietly, focusing on the absolute irony of the day. As I was escorted back to the infusion center, I kept thinking about how much I hated my birthday being in February because Chicago is always so cold. I figured the timing of all of this meant something . . . but I wasn't sure I knew what it was.

My first treatment was scheduled to take eight full hours, so I was given a private room. I didn't think to ask, and no one explained that the first infusion drips are slowed so they can monitor for any allergic reactions. I remember everything about that day, but what stands out to me most was all the beeping sounds from the machines as others were finishing or starting their infusions.

The feeling of cold permeated in the air, right into my veins, and then onto my hands as I held ice packs from fingers to palm, in order to prevent neuropathy. The sloshing, bloated feeling in my stomach caused by both the IV liquids and hydrating all day is a feeling I can never forget. But what will forever be burned into my memory is the fear and helplessness on Matt's face. I was usually the fixer, but on this day, I had no comforting words to make this situation any better. I was just trying to survive.

A slow, flu-like feeling crept up all over my body as soon as my treatment ended and it lingered, giving me a preview of the long movie ahead. I also experienced a strange, disassociated feeling in my brain. I think I managed through that first day okay, but the next two weeks were some of the hardest weeks of my whole journey. I had an adverse reaction to a post-injection that caused a prickling in my body, like a body-buzz high that just continued to intensify until it devolved into a hum of pain. I was prescribed pain killers, but even that couldn't touch the deep aches that were vibrating from my bones. The nausea was so intense, and eating became a challenge. The daytime exhaustion caused by the nighttime insomnia left me in a mental fog. I still had my hair, but every day while showering or brushing, I wondered if this would be the day I pulled out clumps.

I didn't plan to shave my head that day. I wasn't ready; not emotionally, not mentally. But the day I went to pick out my wig, my scalp tingled and my dark blond strands fell into the bathroom sink, just like leaves falling to the ground at the edge of winter. Each falling strand was its own small heartbreak. My body was already letting go, and I couldn't stop it. The wig shop doubled as a hair studio, and the owner had guided many other women before me through this process. I didn't feel ready, but he patiently talked me through the next steps. "How about we just cut it into a pixie cut, and then you can decide what's next," he gently suggested. As he cut my hair shorter and shorter, then finally picked up the razor, the truth settled in. This was real now. Cancer was no longer something I could hide from. I was someone who dealt with life more internally. I tried to muddle through on my own, rarely asking for help. I was often self-conscious about my looks, hiding behind my hair, using makeup as a shield to cover up what I felt were imperfections. Now there was no shield. For the first time in my life, I felt truly exposed.

It was dark in the car as I headed home. I kept touching the soft fuzz left on my head, stealing glances in the rearview mirror. I had asked for a level three on the clippers so I could avoid being fully bald until the rest of my hair fell out. I thought I would break down crying in the privacy of my car, but instead, I felt a strange mix of relief and numbness. Then a pit formed in my stomach. I realized I hadn't talked to Matt or Nolan about when or how I was going to shave my head. I grabbed my phone and texted, "I just wanted to warn you that I shaved my head tonight. I didn't want to scare you when I walked in. Can you prepare Nolan?"

As I parked and got ready to go inside, I wanted to do two opposite things at once—run in to get it over with, and run away to avoid it entirely. I decided to get it over with, so I opened the door and walked in. Matt and Nolan were watching TV in the living room. Matt stood up, walked over, and hugged me. "Why didn't you tell me you were going to shave it today? I could have come." My inner voice screamed, *Because I was afraid. Because I felt exposed. I didn't want to be rejected.*

Nolan stood behind Matt, hesitant and a little unsure. I crouched down and asked him to touch it. "Mommy, it's soft. It doesn't look that bad," he said. I felt a wave of sadness. In trying to protect both them and me from the pain and embarrassment, I had kept them out of this big moment. I hadn't allowed them to grieve with me, to begin the transition from seeing me as healthy to watching me fight cancer. Over the next few days, the last of my hair shed into my hats and scarves, leaving me completely bald. At that time and throughout my treatment, I still felt too vulnerable. I never let my family see me without anything on my head.

At first, the six rounds of chemo didn't sound too bad. I thought, *I can do anything for six days, especially if they are three weeks apart.* What I didn't know then, and what I can hardly think about, even now, is the mental anguish that became impossible to ignore in between my sessions. With each subsequent treatment, I would have less good days and more days where I couldn't move, couldn't eat, couldn't walk down the hall without being breathless. The depression and anxiety that had been my lifelong companions took up residence on either side of me, whispering into my ears that this cancer treatment was going to destroy me; that maybe I couldn't make it through. It took all my strength to convince my mind that while it felt like I was dying, in fact, this poison coursing through my veins, was the very thing that would save my life.

Depression and anxiety had shaped my life in many ways, and along with that shaping, I carried a hefty amount of shame. I had a good life; I didn't have a reason to feel so sad. I felt weak for not being able to pull myself out of this sadness. I had it all; high school popularity, a college education, a supportive family. As I got older, I built a solid career, had many good friends, and married a good and caring husband. From the outside looking in, people considered me to be a likeable, easy going, thoughtful, creative person. But on the inside, I was deeply sad, weird, lonely, and unworthy.

During one depressing winter, I was holed up in my apartment, when I stumbled across a documentary about a stranded whale in a Norwegian bay. The story stirred something raw and unhealed in me, a vulnerable place I hadn't yet found the words for. Separated from his pod, the whale had been adopted by the local town. He swam alongside boats, craving connection, and eventually allowed people to touch him. He seemed to thrive on human attention, and the bay became his home. But the boats that brought him comfort also posed a deadly threat; their propellers could kill him. So, for his protection, the town made it illegal to touch him. People were told to ignore him, even to turn their backs when he approached. The whale, confused and heartbroken, withdrew into loneliness. Watching him, I felt his despair seep through the screen and match my own. I cried deep, aching sobs.

This whale's story didn't end well. He never left the bay to find his lost family or socialize with other whale pods, until one day he was fatally injured by a boat and died lonely and alone. At the time, the whale represented the root of my depression; fear of being rejected, left lonely and alone. Never finding where I belonged. When I revisited the whale again during cancer, he represented the loneliness I felt during treatment. I had a lot of support and help, but only *I* was sick. Only I was facing the rapid decline of my body from the side effects and a premature brush with my mortality.

The loneliness was most pronounced at night, when my body was too tired to keep going, but my mind wouldn't stop and let me rest. I would wake up drenched in sweat caused by hot flashes or over-whelming nausea, or both. I would tiptoe to the bathroom, my son and husband sleeping soundly in the other room, and lie on the floor sick until I could find the strength to crawl back into bed. I was envious of their restful sleep and the normalcy of their lives when they woke up.

As sleep eluded me, my phone became a portal to the inner corners of my mind. Each night I would search the ends of the internet for more and more information on breast cancer. My anxiety was overflowing. My health, my career, my marriage, my ability to be the parent I wanted to be—all of it felt so out of my control. Learning everything I could about my cancer gave me a sense of control I was missing. When I devoured all the medical information I could, I started seeking out videos that spoke to my deeper fear: leaving my family early. I remember watching the ending scene from *American Beauty*. As the main character Lester lays dying, he experiences flashes of beauty in his life in small moments and details. And then he sees his daughter Jane at the door as a teenager, then Jane as a child. I kept imagining Nolan, just in kindergarten, remembering only snippets of his mom and how much she loved him. And then him opening the door as a teenager and me not being able to see him growing into a young man.

As I contemplated mortality, I read so many devastating stories of fellow women who had not made it through this disease. *What if I came out of this alive? Why were these strong, brave women with full lives ahead of them not spared?* One particular lonely night, as these stories and my worries began to overwhelm me and pull me into my dark spiral, I realized that if I was going to actually survive this thing with my body *and* mind intact, I was going to need a different type of support.

I began seeking out support groups on social media, including one focused specifically on my type of breast cancer and another for younger women who were going through or had been through cancer. These women, like me, were often awake at three in the morning, alone in their dark houses, battling nausea, pain, and the heavy weight of loneliness. They shared jokes about the strange things chemo was doing to our bodies. They sent clapping hands and heart emojis to celebrate each other's milestones. And when someone felt ready to give up, on treatment or on life, they stepped in and held her up. In many ways, I felt closer to these women than to people in my day-to-day life. I had found my whales! They helped me survive the darkest nights, reminding me of life's quiet gifts and the wisdom we gain from one another. It was a community that I desperately needed when I believed my only option was to suffer alone.

As chemo wore down my body, the familiar shadows of doubt and depression returned. I couldn't power through on my own anymore. I had to accept help—from my mom, from friends, from family. My mom stepped in completely, pushing aside her own fear to be strong for me. Because when you're a parent, you'll do whatever it takes to help your child survive. She did that for me so I could do the same for Nolan. Without ever asking, other people showed up too. Friends checked in weekly and dropped off meals. My aunts and uncles sent notes and thoughtful gifts. My niece and nephew wore pink ribbons during their games. Matt kept our loved ones updated and received kind words in return. A few close friends even rotated as my chemo companions, sitting with me during long infusions. As much as I dreaded the sickness that followed, I found myself looking forward to those visits; the quiet conversations, the shared stillness, the feeling of not being alone. They helped carry the weight. And in their presence, I felt supported, seen, and deeply grateful.

As I approached my sixth and last chemo, I started to feel a little lighter. I thought I would quit after treatment five, but here I was, at the edge of completing the hardest, longest six months of my life. I did it, in part, because of the community and support I had around me, but I was also secretly proud of my strength to survive something as life changing as cancer. Tears pricked my eyes as I sat in that chemo chair for the last time and then rang the bell, my husband right there next to me. I know not everyone has the privilege of ringing the bell; some people have lifelong chemo treatments, so I was grateful and humbled as the bell rope vibrated in my hands.

I didn't celebrate right away. I still had weeks of side effects ahead of me. But when I learned the tumor had completely shrunk and later, my lumpectomy showed clean margins, I finally had the proof that treatment had worked. I was declared NED. For the first time in my life, I felt strong in my spirit. I had built a supportive community around me, even if I hadn't fully seen it before through the fog of depression. For years, I had carried shame, convinced by my inner voice that I was weak and unworthy. But standing at the end of treatment, I knew there was nothing weak about me. I had beaten cancer!

In the months that followed, life shifted from grayscale to vivid color. Everything felt brighter, more textured, more alive. As I returned to daily routines, at work, at home, and with friends, I felt grounded by gratitude and a renewed sense of joy. I had once believed strength meant holding everything together and hiding the cracks. But cancer stripped that belief away. I couldn't hide the exhaustion, the hair loss, or the fear in my son's eyes. So I stopped trying. I let people in. I allowed myself to be carried. And in that vulnerability, I discovered a deeper strength.

The posttreatment glow faded. Life is hard and I am forever a work in progress. I still manage depression and self-doubt, because like cancer, they don't just go away. They require care and attention. But I have gained something that lifts me above the noise: a wider perspective. I never would have pictured myself as a cancer survivor the day I found the grape-sized lump in my breast. Yet here I am on the other side, and I am proud to say I am a more whole person. It is always in the back of my mind that cancer will return, and while I would never have chosen this particular path, what I know now is how strong I am, and that regardless of what lies ahead, I have what I need to carry on.

AUTHOR BIO

Liz Gerber is a writer, marketer, and mother. As a brand manager, she brings her creativity and strategic mindset to the world of consumer goods and has worked for brands such as LEGO, Sharpie, Coca-Cola, and Hostess.

After her own breast cancer diagnosis in 2022, Liz found strength in storytelling, using words to navigate the emotional and physical challenges of recovery. Her writing has always been personal, and this will be her first writing experience sharing with others. As a contributing author to this anthology, Liz hopes her story reminds others that healing is not just about survival, it's about rediscovering wholeness and purpose.

When she is not writing or working, Liz is a wife and mother, finding joy in family adventures, the great outdoors, and savoring the simple moments of everyday life.

SARAH ZSAK

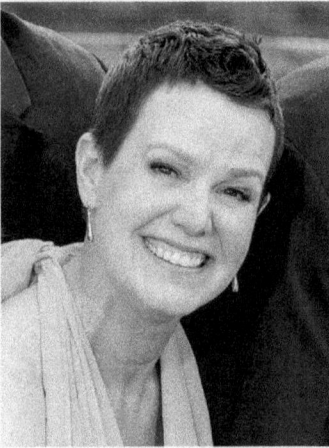

The world seemed to pause, except for the pine branches which blew in the breeze, blocking my view of my son. That's exactly what's going to happen, I thought. My view ends here. I will never get to see him, or any of my children grow up. I won't get to find out what it's like to be old and retired with Neil. I can perhaps best describe it as a feeling of the ultimate FOMO, a gut-wrenching feeling of missing out, on everything. My heart sank as I realized I would never get to see all the love and work for my family come to fruition. I was in utter shock. I guess that's it. That was short. I walked over to pick my son up as soccer ended and felt out of control. What did anything matter?

TIME WITH MY BABIES

I couldn't believe it, and the doctor couldn't either. "Come back in six months," he directed nonchalantly, "and if you can get the mammogram from your miscarriage at thirty-seven, it would be good to have for comparison." His voice sounded detached, as if he was absentmindedly selecting kung pao chicken off a menu for the fifth time for dinner, his eye contact with me brief. He and the tech, whose eyes in contrast to the doctors, seemed worried, towered over me in our powder-room-sized stall, the curtain mostly open. I wondered what the older ladies in neighboring stalls were thinking. I sat dutifully in my gown, which stubbornly refused to stay closed, mentally ticking off everything else I needed to do that day. In many ways, I couldn't blame the doctor. As if I was trying to avoid wasting his time I stated quickly, "I've been told I just have lumpy, bumpy breasts." Which was true. I had no family history of breast cancer. I was an active mom of four young kids. I had no other symptoms besides a subtle change in the shape of my right breast over the last few months. And for a variety of reasons, I hadn't been able to get this mammogram until May. I had been told it would be a diagnostic mammogram, but it was not. As it turned out, other symptoms lurked below the surface, where the naked eye couldn't see. What the radiologist discovered that day was a bright white blizzard of cancer cells in my right breast, apparently obscured by dense breast tissue. In this pressurized time-driven healthcare system, our conversation lasted no more than seven minutes. Probably five.

I felt nothing, really. No concern. I just looked at my watch and planned my next task for the day, in order to maximize efficiency. *It's always been benign before* was the thought that cycled through my head. I had dealt with benign tumors called fibroadenomas in my twenties and thirties, and when I asked, was told they did not increase my breast cancer risk, which I now know was a terrible inaccuracy. As it turns out, most women who develop breast cancer have no family history of it. Alcohol consumption and hormone use (e.g. fertility medications or birth control) increase our risk, particularly before our first childbirth. So I did have a number of significant risk factors which I obediently reported onto my medical history forms, but they never translated into any action. When I turned forty in 2022, I was asked at my physical by my previous primary care doctor only if I had family history of breast cancer. I did not, and was told I should start mammograms at fifty. Not long after, unbeknownst to me, guidance was changed to forty.

Many emails, phone calls, and lots of legwork later, persistence paid off, and I was ready to take a CD of my comparison mammogram from age thirty-seven to the hospital. I replied all to a long email chain of managers and medical staff I had accumulated in my quest, reporting that I would drop the CD off that day. On the CD sleeve I wrote my name, date of birth, the doctor's name, and "FOR COMPARISON." I repeated all this information to the woman at the front desk, whose raised brows and pursed lips betrayed the fact that I may have been placed into the overreactor category of patients. I gave her the CD and filed out with my seven-year-old in her leotard, just in time to make it to her gymnastics class.

A couple months later, I noticed a message from my gynecologist pop up in my patient portal. She was following up on my mammogram and wanted to remind me the radiologist would like my comparison CD. I hit reply immediately and wrote in short sentences that I had delivered the CD nearly two months before, but had not heard back. "I figured no news was good news . . ." I typed then hit send. "No, they are supposed to write an addendum," she messaged back. So, I added another email to the already miles long email chain to my local hospital. They said they would look into it.

The next day, I received a voicemail from the hospital admitting that my mammogram CD had indeed been lost. They had found the CD and the mammogram coordinator would be calling me. The manager sent me an email just over an hour later with the same information. Two minutes later, the mammogram coordinator also left a voicemail saying I needed to come back in as soon as possible for another mammogram. I could read between the lines. Obviously a doctor had compared my old mammogram taken at age thirty-seven with the one I'd just had, and something didn't look right. I quickly returned to the hospital, got back into the tiny booth clad in the gown that refused to stay shut, this time meeting with a different radiologist after a diagnostic mammogram.

His face was drawn, his eyes concerned. "You have breast cancer," he told me.

While I knew this was the moment that everything in my life would change, I couldn't picture exactly how. I didn't know quite what we were dealing with; I just knew I was young, I was healthy, and in shape. I trusted modern medicine and I trusted my body. If I was really honest, I had been through so much in my lifetime, a breast cancer diagnosis felt like nothing compared to multiple miscarriages or the medical issues we'd experienced with our children. It was unsettling, yes, but I was just glad that it would be me dealing with this disease and that my kids had been spared.

I managed the next steps in stride and, to be honest, I mom pretty hard—anytime I got a chance to stop moving, it felt like a break. I remember nearly falling asleep on the biopsy table waiting for the doctor to take samples. Frankly, for a little bit there, it looked like all this was just going to offer me a free boob job and an opportunity for a nice long break from responsibilities!

It didn't help that the same local hospital seemed used to the still-scary-but-slower-growing forms of breast cancer found to be more common in older women. "You've got time," I was told by a medical staffer on the phone. "This didn't get here overnight." While reassuring, I can now say that was very bad advice. I've since learned that breast cancer is a constellation of related diseases, with some being significantly more aggressive than others. The local hospital just didn't seem set up for the urgency and critical timeline of this. My kind of breast cancer was relatively rare, and I'm not sure how many of the 4 percent of us they'd seen.

Five days later, I offered to take my older daughter and her sweet friend back-to-school shopping. The words "breast cancer" were on my mind, but I was still trying to piece together what they meant for me. We were at a teen consignment shop, and I saw a pair of surprisingly-practical office dress boots. I reached for them, then stopped myself. I had been so busy running the kids back and forth to activities, getting ready to start a new school year, and just trying to keep up, that I hadn't really thought about the fact that I might not be able to go back to work because of my diagnosis. I stroked the soft leather with my fingertips and an even darker thought made its way into my mind: *Some people do still die from cancer.* As the girls piled up shorts and tops at the register I had the stark realization that maybe, I actually was really sick, and might have to completely change my lifestyle. My usual mentality of "everything will be fine" started to waver as I began to understand that I might not actually be able to control the outcome of cancer, no matter how mentally and physically strong I was. I looked at my daughter again, and felt a rush of emotion and the depth of the moment come over me as she continued laughing with her friend. It was as if I was at a crossroads, and one path led me down the dark road of despair, while the other one, even though I couldn't see the end, felt more like life and light. I knew that I had very few choices when it came to cancer, but I had a choice right then and there, about which path I was going to take. I picked up the boots and marched over to the cash register and paid for them immediately. I had a long hard road to walk. I was going to need these boots. *Dear God, please help me stay with my family.*

As a new school year started, work began, so I drove my kids to day care and YMCA day camp. In my mind, the question of what on earth was happening with my body was tumbling around like the never-ending loads of laundry I piled into the dryer day after day. My kids popped out of the van sunroof while we waited in the drop-off line. K-LOVE radio played some of our favorite songs, and I was able to convince myself that all was right with the world. As I drove away from camp, I waved goodbye to my kids as I moseyed along a particularly beautiful stretch of country road. I noticed how beautiful the stretch was, dappled with sunshine allowing for peeks of gorgeous views. I had been traveling this route with my children every summer for years. And then suddenly a thought hit me, *Will this be my last time?* It filled me, for the first time, with a sense of grief for the loss of our beautiful life together, for the idyllic existence they didn't know was about to end.

The question of how serious this illness actually was, was answered when my first pathology report came in. I opened the letter and was shocked it showed eight out of nine possible points registered on the aggression scale. The world stopped as terror rolled over me like a dark fog, choking out my hope for a future with my children. *Could the report be right? Was it possible that I did not indeed have time, and that this thing was growing fast?* I didn't want to tell my husband Neil. He loved me more than anything. I so wanted to protect him from this news, to let him focus on the dream job he had just landed and all the emotions that came with that. But he deserved to be aware of the worst and together we would hope for the best.

When he got home from his new job, I asked him to join me out on the deck. For some reason I laughed with discomfort when I showed him the report. He was stunned. We decided we needed to seek a second opinion from a top-notch research institution, and in our area that often means Johns Hopkins. We are fortunate to have a facility like that within driving distance. I started to pray harder. *Please God, let me stay with my husband and babies,* was all I could manage.

When I called Hopkins that Tuesday, I was frustrated, but not surprised, to hear the next appointment with a breast surgeon was over two and a half weeks away. That is a lifetime when you are trying to stop a fast-growing cancer, but I booked it. That Friday night at exactly 9:09 p.m., I was brushing my teeth when I was surprised to see an alert pop up on my phone, asking me to confirm my new appointment. It was for Tuesday at 9 a.m. with a Hopkins breast surgeon! My heart jumped and I yelled for my husband through toothpaste foam, "I need to run upstairs to my laptop, right away!" I hit confirm faster than I had responded to anything in my life.

Monday morning I got a call from the breast surgeon's office. The scheduler said they were not sure what happened, but there was already another patient scheduled for the 9 a.m. Tuesday appointment, and she had been waiting for weeks. I pleaded with her. "I have four young kids here at home. My cancer is growing quickly." My voice caught on a sob that was trying to escape the back of my throat. After a moment of silence, she sighed and promised she'd talk with the surgeon. I stared at my children's artwork on the fridge and wondered if I should believe her. It was my first day teaching in two classes, so I had to woman up and put breast cancer in a box in the back of my mind.

The scheduler, Ms. McGraw, called back, much to my surprise. "Dr. Sogunro has agreed to see you at 9:45 a.m." They had decided to use less time than they normally allowed for a transition interval before starting surgery that day. "Oh my goodness, thank you!" I sobbed through my tears as I collapsed with relief. The next day, as my husband and I were called back to the exam room, the nurse explained that they didn't know what happened, or why I had gotten that alert. They'd never had a glitch in their system like that before. The IT department was looking into it. "I think you better ask a higher power!" I smiled as she shut the door, leaving me in the exam room with my husband.

I learned that the "Holy Trinity" of breast cancer was: breast surgeon, medical oncologist, and radiation oncologist, and I would meet them in that order. Our Hopkins breast surgeon referred us to a Hopkins medical oncologist, who squeezed us in the very next week. The big day of the appointment came, and Neil left early from his new job so we could meet in the parking lot to embrace, before entering what turned out to be the wrong building. A kind staffer pointed at a wall and tried to give us directions, but our heads were swirling as we entered a second building then a third, with no sign of the medical oncology department. My eyes burned with tears and I was filled with fear as I looked at my watch and realized with dismay that my appointment was starting. Neil is not one to embarrass himself and doesn't like to stand out generally. Yet, for me, in that moment, he was so brave. "Let's run," I shouted, already out of breath, and we took off like maniacs. We weren't just running for my life I realized, but for our life together, and for our children to have a mom. I pushed myself to go faster by directing my thoughts silently to my kids and my husband, who was sweating beside me, *I will do everything I can to stay with you. I will do everything I can to stay with you.* Breathlessly, we checked in, panting and wiping sweat from our worried brows. We clasped hands, praying we weren't too late. There were no sweeter words than the front desk receptionist telling us "You're fine" as we made our excuses for our tardiness. We hoped someday, we'd hear "You're fine" again.

It turned out I had an 8.7 cm tumor (basically my entire right breast), which had probably spread to lymph nodes in my armpit and center of my chest, if not further. This made me at least stage 3, the last stage before incurable. All I could think as they explained to me that I would definitely be starting chemo was *I have four young kids.*

There are so many hoops to jump through between initial diagnosis and starting treatment. The medical oncologist we saw that day had been right, this was the hardest part; not knowing what we were dealing with, and then waiting for results. In truth, I didn't do much waiting; I did a lot of waging war. I held a vivid vision of myself as a general on a cliff, overlooking the smoldering valley below, opening a double scroll map on some flat rock face. I saw myself pondering plans with my trusty lieutenant Neil listening attentively over my shoulder. I envisioned myself some kind of nice version of Genghis Khan, sending my scouts out everywhere.

Advocating for and at these testing appointments became like my new job. At one point I was heartened to hear that there were two exclamation points behind the stat in one of my test orders. The tests were scary, not only because of the potential results, but also in the moment, because I'd never done them before and didn't know what to expect. I kept wondering if a test would all be over relatively quickly—would it be fairly routine, like a CT scan which mainly involved ignoring the false sensation that I'd accidentally wet my pants, or would it be very difficult, like an MRI? Trying to hold as still as I could in order to provide the best result for over thirty minutes while I was being sent into a tunnel that sounded like it was being jackhammered was nearly impossible. Despite the hardships, I was so grateful for access to cutting edge medical care, and the ability to check another box off my long diagnostic list. But my heart would race as I would try to mentally prepare for any IV placement gone awry, strange substance to drink within a specific timeframe, cup to pee in, order to remove my clothes, or position they asked me to hold. I would gear up to ignore the sights/sounds/smells turning my stomach. In an effort to find peace and comfort, I began to picture myself sitting not on a starkly cold medical table, but instead, I visualized myself sitting in the palm of God's hand. As machines would move my body into some tube or another on a tray-like bed, I would picture I was lying on the chest of Jesus who was holding and protecting me. Making the long drives to and from appointments, I would often listen to the piano version of "Never Will" by Life.Church Worship. Even in the middle of traffic, it reminded me that God would never let me go.

The PET scan was the most critical test for me because this would determine how far the cancer had spread, and if it had gone to any of the big-four incurable areas that breast cancer can spread to: brain, bone, lung, or liver. If it had, that would mean I was metastatic. I felt the lymph nodes in my neck nearly every day, searching for swelling that could mean my cancer was marching onward towards my brain.

Given the size of the tumor and the fact that the MRI had shown it had likely already spread to lymph nodes in the center of my chest and in my armpit, my medical oncologist was realistic. I'll never forget her words. "I've seen HER2 cancers *as extensive as yours* with no distant spread. I've also seen women with a tiny spot of HER2 and it's already everywhere." This did not sound promising. I've never prayed so hard in my life. I begged God, *Please, if there's a choice, let me stay and raise my babies.*

The day of my PET, I got my four kids up and ready as usual. As soon as the elementary and middle school buses left, I dropped my youngest off at day care and made the hour-plus drive north. I had three appointments over the course of eight hours, so I was periodically returning to my van, which I had parked in the hospital parking lot, under the trees. I sat inside the van, windows rolled down and sunroof open, allowing the fresh air to wash over me as I processed what was happening and prayed. I basked in the dappled sunlight and let it soothe me, listening to the tree's leaves swaying in the wind. I felt so scared as I clung to my prayer cards. *Please God, help me and my family stay together.* I prayed, over and over again.

The PET result came back via my phone, surprisingly quickly. It had only been an hour and twenty minutes. I had been trying to focus on the trees and concentrate on my breathing. I felt the world stop turning as I clumsily punched an index finger onto the screen of my phone. The result took my breath away. I clasped my hand to my mouth and had to crawl from the driver's seat to the center, flattened out between the two car seats. I began to sob. It was shockingly beautiful. No distant spread was seen! I was still in stage 3. Right there, in that parking lot, the mercy of being spared and knowing God had heard all the prayers we had prayed at all hours of the day and night, overwhelmed me. In gratitude I promised God, *I can do better before you call me home.* I knew I could be so much more intentional about how I spent this borrowed time. I could help others more and try to live up to being "the hands and feet" of God. I could spend more of this gift of time on what really mattered. Not on outer accomplishments and pointless gold stars, but on love and relationships.

The day came when we knew we had to tell our children. I'll admit, we weren't pros at this, I mean, who is? To this day, when we announce a family meeting to our kids, a flash of fear sometimes shows on their faces. We lined them up on the couch and I sat across from them in what we usually call "the birthday chair"—the place where you unwrap gifts—my husband by my side. I offhandedly noticed my older son needed a haircut. They looked so carefree, and I fought back tears at the thought of taking that away from them. "Mommy wanted to let you all know that I have something called cancer. I'm getting treatment. I might be going to the doctor a lot. At times I might be tired and not feel good. But you all will be well taken care of." They looked surprised but didn't say much. My sweet oldest, who rarely makes any trouble, showed me just how hard this news was.

Neil had been giving me space as I laid in bed that evening, then came in to offer me dinner. He looked exhausted and told me that when he had walked into the family room he saw books, couch cushions, and pillows thrown everywhere. He found our oldest, Leta, trashing the space, which was completely out of character for her. Understandably overwhelmed with emotion, not long after, my poor girl came to my bedside crying. She was afraid I was going to die.

Finally, we were only waiting on one thing to start treatment. An appointment. Early, every day, I took up my position at the kitchen table, phone in hand, and called the same eight numbers, checking to see if there had been any cancellations so I could move the triple biopsy appointment earlier. One staffer told me, "Your name has been everywhere!" My goal was to start treatment within one month of diagnosis. I had booked an aspirational first-chemo appointment for the one day before the one month mark, a Friday. If I didn't start treatment that day, I would not only miss my goal but would have to wait two additional days for the weekend. I was acutely aware that things could spread from stage 3 to terminal, any day.

The morning of my deadline, I saw there had been no update on the pending lynchpin results, which were needed before we could go ahead with treatment. I ballparked a 20 percent chance that we would start that day, which didn't seem promising. My medical oncologist was very cautious and had said she wanted to wait for all the results before beginning chemo. Yet, my husband had taken off work and we decided to make the hour-plus journey to the hospital, if for nothing else, we figured we could at least talk with the doctor and advocate. I checked in, not sure what the appointment was for. They called my name, and my husband and I followed, past the turn to the doctor's office. My heart sped up. *Could it be? What was straight ahead?* We passed some beige medical recliners and intricate IV pumps, and then a nurse's station behind glass. Suddenly our nurse stopped and whisked back a curtain. Like a world-class magician, she revealed an incredible sight. I froze. "Do I get to start today?" My nurse smiled at my question, and when she answered yes, I wept with relief. All this work, all this fighting, and I'd done it! I was finally going to get the treatment that could help keep me around for my kids. I was the happiest sick girl in the world as I climbed into that chemo chair.

It didn't take long for my side effects to really hit. One family tradition we've always tried to maintain is family dinner time. On Chemo

Day 7, I spent most of the day resting, and my husband grilled burgers as a treat. One of the kids was ill and I was concerned about residual germs, but it broke my heart to miss another dinner with my family. So I sat at a table in the next room with the plate my husband made me, in an attempt to feel like we were together. I took one bite and gagged. It tasted like pennies, and immediately a wave of nausea came over me. Big tears rolled down my cheeks. My family was so gentle and understanding as I gave away my burger and went downstairs to my bed.

After a few weeks of chemo, the inevitable happened: my hair started falling out. It's not like I had ever considered my hair to be my crowning glory—it was mousy brown and fairly thin, but the fact that it was falling out in clumps was just proof that I looked as bad on the outside as I felt on the inside. Even worse was the reaction my youngest experienced to my newly bald head. The morning my husband shaved it, my normally affectionate three-year-old was afraid of me. "It's ok," I tried to assure him. "It's something new." My heart cracked as Colton started to back up, crying. I can't blame him. His world was turned upside down, and one of the most basic facts—what his parent looked like—was pulled out from under him. My cell phone no longer recognized my face and refused to unlock. *Who am I now?* was all I could think.

When I first learned how serious my diagnosis was, I envisioned our family experiencing indescribable amounts of stress and isolation. I saw myself lashing out at everyone around me and then feeling ashamed. I pictured Neil at his breaking point, all of which scarring the kids for life. Yet that is not at all what happened. I'm embarrassed to say I'm not sure exactly how all the help started, but I know it began with our church. Our wonderful priest, Father Mike, came by the house and said simply, "We are your church family. Anything you need: lawn mowed, meals delivered, you name it, we are here for you." The church women's group prayed for us and cooked for us, 219 times to date, to be exact. When our younger daughter Lucy really wanted to get to Sunday School, which felt like an impossibility, a church director put together a signup for taking her to church.

Our kids' teammates, coaches, and dance friends helped transport our children to and from their activities, and family members as well as new friends jumped in too. These were incredible folks who, sometimes after a long day's work, still found the time and energy to help our children stay on their teams and keep their lives as normal as possible, as opposed to being stuck at home with a sick mom. Any piece of normal we could get at that time was a gift, as was the lesson that bad things can happen, but there are many kind people who are available to help. I am so grateful that my children have experienced God's love firsthand, in this way. I rarely went out of my way to help people before my diagnosis, but now I see how absolutely critical it is. I learned through cancer that helping others is one of the most important things we can do in this life.

For me, chemo side effects were very cyclical, and so became predictable, and we were able to successfully move my son's fourth birthday and Christmas to days where I felt almost human. I was able to time going out for a run (sometimes ridiculously slowly) throughout my illness, unless it was medically forbidden. It was important to keep my heart healthy because cardiac toxicity was one of the things that could stop my treatment. Often on the last stretch, I would visualize carrying one of my children over my shoulder to safety, spurring me on.

As weeks rolled into months, the roller coaster caused by cancer continued when I discovered a mysterious new lump in my right armpit. I noticed it one beautiful Sunday morning as my family was enjoying much-needed quality time together. I had promised them I would do everything I possibly could to stick around for them, so I forced myself to phone the oncologist on call. He directed me to drive to downtown Baltimore for oncology urgent care. It was so hard leaving all my kids as they happily jumped on the trampoline in the sunshine.

Oncology urgent care turned out to be the upper floor of a medical high rise. It felt like a ghost town on a Sunday, the dimly lit corridors and abandoned equipment making it seem incredibly spooky. The hospital rooms were semi-private, and as I entered, I noticed a woman who would be my new roommate, already in the other bed. Our eyes locked as I passed by. Hers were bright blue and I could tell we were kindred spirits. She was maybe fifteen years older than me, thin with chemo-shortened hair; her muddy duck boots set neatly by her bed, suggesting she had been enjoying the outdoors before whatever had sent her here. As I settled into my bed, it struck me that one of the most tragic things about cancer, or any major illness really, is how it steals people's ability to do things they love. I sighed, wondering how lunch was going, wishing I was the one who was at home preparing it for my family. Eight hours, a CT scan, and an ultrasound later, the lump was diagnosed as an infection, much to my relief.

Dealing with cancer aged me thirty years. Medical professionals and staff usually just assumed I had time to talk when they called, but a little background kid cacophony or sneaking in "I'm driving my daughter to ballet class, can I call you back?" sometimes helped get my particular reality across. Some medical offices unilaterally made appointments that would never work for the schedule of a parent of young children. The sobering reality hit my husband and I one morning when we decided to take an opportunity to go out for lunch after an appointment, even though it was just 11:15 a.m. We caught the early crowd at an Outback Steakhouse and as we looked around, realized basically every other occupied table had a couple, twenty-five to forty-five years older than we were. I figured they were probably also between medical appointments. "What are we doing here?" we wondered to each other as we opened the overwhelmingly large menus "Why are we here decades early?"

As I rang the bell for what I thought would be my final chemo treatment, my mind immediately jumped toward the next step; a double mastectomy and lymph node removal. Outwardly, my tumor had responded dramatically to four months of aggressive chemotherapy. My once-diseased breast had returned to normal softness, and I was able to return to my previous smaller bra size. The surgical procedures themselves were blurs of pains and drains, but the real agony was in the results. Four small spots of cancer had remained in what the surgeon had removed. Those cells had developed resistance to the chemotherapy, meaning a higher risk of cancer striking again. This so-called residual disease sorted me, Harry Potter style, into the "you might want to start getting your affairs in order" group.

With the rug pulled out from under me, I met with my medical oncologist to talk about my residual disease results. She typed, and I noticed the click of her nails as I peeked over her shoulder and was able to decipher her notes. She had written "T3N1M0 now T1N1Mx" meaning: big tumor, node-positive, not metastatic, had become: small tumor, node positive, and unknown metastatic. The sight of the x made my breath catch in my throat. My doctor was hedging her bets on whether or not I was now stage 4 and incurable. I was told to look for any new persistent pain (bone), shortness of breath (lung), changes in vision/dizziness (brain). *Please God, no. Let me stay with my babies.*

With residual disease, it was back to chemo, a less aggressive but longer one, plus a clinical trial. This time it would be for forty-two weeks, with the aptly-named Dr. Santa-Maria. It was February 2024 and we called it the "chemo till Christmas" plan, which seemed impossibly far away.

One positive of cancer it took me awhile to see was the long-time horizon. Cancer tends to be a marathon and not a sprint. Even "fast" cases take weeks to months. So there can be time to think and course correct. As more weeks turned into even more months, we chipped away at the fourteen new chemo cycles, and I had time to reconsider my priorities. We added thirty daily proton radiation treatments on top of the chemo and clinical trial. And on the additional two-hour plus daily drives to and from the hospital, I started to realize some things. I learned about a word, antifragile, coined by Nassim Nicholas Taleb, which referred essentially to next-level resilience. The idea was not just to make it through difficulty and return to what had been, but to see what is possible now, because of that difficulty. So I started considering what could be made better from the difficulties my family was facing. For me, one way was to prioritize how I spent my time better. Not on trying to achieve what popular culture defines as success, but on real, lasting success: showing love to other people by lending a hand or spending quality time with them.

A friend of mine who lost her husband to cancer said there were things she wished they'd done together before he passed. Rachel's advice to all was, "Take the trip, see the movie, spend the time. You never know when you won't get later." I knew she'd "been there," so

I trusted her. I stopped postponing, and we took five family trips in eight months: Maryland's Eastern Shore with CaringOn, a farm cabin in rural Virginia, the total solar eclipse in Lake Erie and New York, Justin's Beach House in Delaware, and Little Pink Houses of Hope in Tahoe. We went sailing, twice. I knew there was a chance we'd never have the opportunity again, and that I had a responsibility to my family to grab on to as many special moments as I could. As I watched my children run through fields at the foothills of the Blue Ridge Mountains, I knew I had finally made the right decision by prioritizing what really mattered. I was choosing the things that would actually last, even into the next life.

Not long after, I got CT scan results that rocked my world. It was two days after my older daughter turned twelve and the day before my older son turned ten. I had dropped him off at an evening soccer clinic and was sitting in the shade of a large conifer, watching the kids play from a distance. I opened my medical portal to find new results, as I often did. I was not expecting any surprises since I was still in active treatment. Yet, there it was. The devastating news I had been terrified of for so long. As I clicked open on the report, I tried to make the letters into words, the words into sentences, and the sentences to make sense. Everything I'd been fearing and trying to outrun swirled around then trapped me.

Two new lung nodules. Lungs. One of the four common places for breast cancer spread when you progress from early-stage breast cancer (1-3) to terminal (stage 4). The world seemed to pause, except for the pine branches which blew in the breeze, blocking my view of my son. *That's exactly what's going to happen*, I thought. *My view ends here. I will never get to see him, or any of my children grow up. I won't get to find out what it's like to be old and retired with Neil.* I can perhaps best describe it as a feeling of the ultimate FOMO, a gut-wrenching feeling of missing out, on everything. My heart sank as I realized I would never get to see all the love and work for my family come to fruition. I was in utter shock. *I guess that's it. That was short.* I walked over to pick my son up as soccer ended and felt out of control. *What did anything matter?* I forced my way into a conversation between a nice mom and the coach, basically demanding that they acknowledge my son Wyatt's upcoming birthday. This was the inflection point. A threshold had been crossed. I felt everything shift. Nothing would ever be the same again. Hope faded.

I had created worst-case scenario plans, which I began to put into action when I was able to think again. They mainly involved trying to hire people to fill in the gaps I'd leave: babysitters, house cleaners, a driver for the kids, and getting everyone more involved in support groups at Wellness House of Annapolis. Because my cancer was so aggressive and fast growing, I would likely only have up to two years left. And there was no guarantee about the quality of that time.

Then I was shocked to start having more consistent pain in my ribs and sternum, which is one of the major signs of bone spread. Or, according to my wonderful radiation oncologists Drs. LaVigne and Wright, it could be related to all the radiation. I desperately hoped they were right. A bone scan was added to my follow up CT for lungs. I lived like I was dying.

The summer ended and it was time for my repeat CT scan and bone scan. Everyone I knew was praying. I walked into the CT scan room that September day filled with trepidation. A year ago I'd done the same thing with the PET scan initial diagnosis. *Please God, help me and my family stay together a little longer.* If there were more nodules, or they were bigger, my goose was likely cooked.

The results came in while I was putting gas in the minivan. I didn't even pull away from the pump to give the next person a space, I just sat there, dumbfounded. Again and again, I read the same line across the report. "No abnormality seen." In this September's CT: nothing. Nada. Zero lymph nodes were too large this time. There was no mention of spots anywhere, just slightly more right lung shadowing, which was consistent with radiation scarring, typically on a delayed timeline just like mine. I was stunned. The bone scan was clear too! It was God's mercy, our prayers had been heard. *This is amazing love.* I was flooded with gratitude for another chance and renewed my vow to try to remember how short life really is and what it's really about, like helping others and prioritizing love, ahead of my last day on Earth.

Today I'm still in the thick of things and trying to make sense of everything. So much has happened on this journey that I can't explain. As one of my favorite songs by Hope Darst says, "After everything I've seen, how can I not believe?" All my little human mind can state for sure is that we are not alone. God sees us, hears us, and helps us.

Not yet a survivor, I am still a warrior and in a new clinical trial. I hope even though the statistics for this trial are so good, I am able to hold on to the gift of the lessons—to be sure I'm prioritizing the right things each moment. Important? Helping other people. Showing love. Spending time together because you may never get another chance. Unimportant? Trying to "win" the kid and career game. Spending time on things you won't even remember in two years. I recently heard cancer described as a severe blessing, and that rings true.

How will it end? No human knows. I'm working on trusting that God loves my children and my husband even more than I do, and knows what's best for us all. I heard before, "If you focus on the wound, you'll continue to hurt. If you focus on the lesson, you'll continue to grow," and I would add to that, "If you focus on the opportunity, you'll use this to become a better version of yourself."

ABOUT THE AUTHOR

Sarah Zsak is a speech-language pathologist (SLP) and mom to four beautiful children. After serving in the Peace Corps in Bolivia, she married her high school sweetheart Neil. She was diagnosed with an aggressive stage 3 breast cancer in August 2023, the day after her steadfast husband started his challenging dream job. Her kids were eleven, nine, seven, and three-years-old at the time. Fortunately, Sarah and her family have been blessed with an avalanche of help from their church Holy Family Catholic Church, as well as community, friends, and family.

Believing she has been spared so far for some purpose, Sarah was taught through cancer that love and relationships are the only things that matter in the end. Whole-heartedly Catholic, she feels all religions should be revered for driving us toward that same positive interconnectedness. Sarah believes she should serve as a witness for the miracles and signs she has personally experienced and the blessings in her life.

Thinking about and facilitating communication and human connection is a passion for Sarah. She enjoys being an adjunct professor at her alma mater University of Maryland, College Park, and a small-business owner with a boutique private speech therapy practice, Terrapin Speech Institute. Sarah practices part-time for the local school system at a Catholic school and a Christian school. She is a member of the American Speech-Language-Hearing Association (ASHA) and an ASHA ACE Award Recipient. She authored the article "Should I Use My Own Children as Therapy Models?" published in the ASHA Leader in 2020. She was a reviewer for the manuscript of telepractice guidebook for SLPs published by Plural Publishing in 2022. Sarah is PROMPT, Lidcombe Program, Orofacial Myology, and PECS trained.

After completing fifteen months of conventional breast cancer treatment as well as an investigational treatment through Johns Hopkins Hospital, Sarah is currently in a clinical trial for a cancer vaccine through Maryland Oncology Hematology. She prays she is prioritizing the right thing in choosing to write about this journey, and wants to help inspire and offer hope to others who are on parallel journeys. She hopes that fear of leaving her kids and spouse can serve as a doorway to compassion for others in a similar predicament.

Sarah would like to thank all the amazing heroes who rode in to rescue her family from this dark and daunting maze, her fantastic medical team, her strong and supportive children Leta, Wyatt, Lucy, and Colton, and her incredible husband Neil. She would also like to thank hopedarst.com for permission to use their lyric. You can learn more about Sarah at her website sites.google.com/terrapinspeechinstitute.com/tsi. When she is able, Sarah enjoys running and gardening at her home in the US, near Annapolis.

ANDREA RALLS

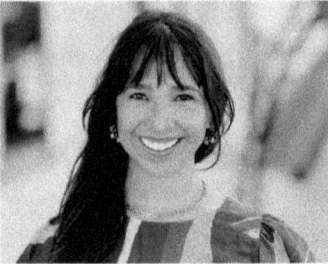

I stood up, albeit unsteadily, and made the final decision: Cancer was not going to get the final say. It was just a chapter in the story of my life, but how that story was told was entirely up to me.

TRUTH IN LOVE

Paralyzed, I fell to my knees on my living room floor, wailing; in that moment, I surrendered everything to God, because I had no other choice. The same three worship songs were on repeat as I sobbed into the carpet, "You have to take this from me, God. I can't do it again." I had followed the plan and stuck to it; I couldn't understand the why or how cancer had resurfaced. The first time, it had been in my breast. It started with a lump, which is easy to dismiss in the haze of postpartum changes. But something nudged me to ask, to follow through. And now I knew: the cancer had been there all along, quietly growing, waiting. If I hadn't been pregnant, it might have stayed hidden for years. Pregnancy didn't just bring new life—it unearthed something dark in me that would have gone unnoticed. This baby growing in me unknowingly pulled danger into the light. My son saved me.

That was the first time. This time, it was in my spine and chest area. Because the cancer had spread to other parts of my body, it was considered late-stage or metastatic. To the medical community, there was no cure; instead, their new focus was only to prolong life. *There is no coming back from this*, I realized as I put my shaking hands over my heart. The verdict, based on medical opinion, felt final. Cancer was going to be my story, and I had finished the book long before I was ready.

With my first cancer diagnosis, there was a treatment plan that included an end date. I could tick the days off the calendar as I went through chemo and subsequent surgeries. Every day was another day closer to being finished. This time was different. There would be no end date or time frame to box in the treatment plan. I was expected to live in uncertainty for the rest of my life. I wasn't sure what would kill me first: the cancer or the not knowing.

Yet, even as my tears kept falling, something inside me shifted. This cancer might have returned, but I didn't have to let it dictate my story. My eyes landed on a photo of my son and family; I was reminded, even in the midst of such devastating news, that I still carried dreams in my heart. There was too much life left in me to lose it all. I had too much love to give and receive.

Ideas began to flood my clearing mind, not just about treatments or appointments, but about healing at every level. I already knew what it took to survive physically, because I had done it once. This time, I wouldn't be flailing in the dark, because I knew what to do. I'd learned to face cancer with light, intention, and faith. And because of that, I knew I wasn't just going to survive, I felt very definite about that. As I wiped my face and drew in a few ragged breaths I felt a presence of peace all around me as I considered the idea that maybe I was being presented with an opportunity to step into something more profound. As I remained in the stillness, my heart knew that my diagnosis was not to be managed alone; I had a supernatural partner on my side and we had one common goal: for me to heal.

I stood up, albeit unsteadily, and made the final decision: Cancer was not going to get the final say. It was just a chapter in the story of my life, but how that story was told was entirely up to me.

"God, I can't do this without You," I finally prayed. My heart lifted in total surrender, and in that moment, I handed over my pain and my unsure future, for the second time. I knew my strength had limits, but I was not operating in my strength alone. I was walking a path, hand in hand with my Creator.

* * *

As I surveyed what needed to be done over the next few weeks, I decided that my feet would not hit the floor until after I gave thanks for another day. I met the morning with a strong conviction that with God, nothing is impossible. Deep in my heart, I believed that there was no sickness He could not heal, no disease He could not cure, and no fight He could not win.

But while I was able to meet my mornings with strength and faith, my belief would begin to wane as the darkness of night took over. For many of those first nights after the diagnosis I felt like I was falling. I moved through our evening routines in a fog, my chest tight with the weight of words I couldn't yet believe. *My cancer is metastatic.* At the dinner table, tears pooled just behind my eyes, pressing forward, demanding to be released as I wondered, *Who would make sure my son ate his vegetables if I wasn't there?* Filled with worry as I put him to bed on those nights, I would buckle under the pain of thinking about who would sing to him if I was gone. Compelled to make sure he remembered the sound of my voice, I would sing an extra round of "Hush Little Baby," while rocking him in the fading twilight. As I sat there in the quiet of the night, watching him sleep, I thought about my husband, his dad. He was everything a father should be, but I couldn't help but believe there were spaces in my son's life only a mother could fill. I felt as empty in those moments as I expected my absence would be for them. I would press my cheek to his cheek, allowing my breathing to follow his rhythm, praying over him with every inhale and exhale. Slowly, my panic would ease—it was not gone, but it softened. Our energy was connected, and we were in sync. I held him closely, as our hearts were connected. It was moments of stillness like these that I would return to again and again when panic and fear of our future would loom heavy.

* * *

Growing up, I had always believed that getting pregnant was a natural part of being a woman. However, it did not come easily for us. After five years of trying, we knew that in vitro fertilization was the most likely option for growing our family. Many months and many shots later, we were ecstatic to find out we were pregnant! Everything was new: new pregnancy symptoms, a new body, and a new baby—and a hard spot on my breast. As I dutifully learned the things I needed to do and be as I began my motherhood journey, I learned my breasts would experience changes during my pregnancy, but as I ran my fingers over the hard spot, I decided it was worth mentioning to my doctor on my next visit. Unsurprisingly, he wasn't worried and just told me to "keep an eye on it."

Six weeks later, it was time to meet my sweet boy.

Several lactation consultants visited us throughout our hospital stay working to ensure an appropriate latch. I pointed out the spot multiple times and was assured that lumps in the breast were "the norm" when my milk came in. My husband and I carried on with all the first days of parenting and newborn things while I also recovered from an arduous birth. Three days later, it was time to go home, which was a long-awaited transition from twenty-four-seven support to parenting all alone. The next three months were like all the other new parent experiences filled with sleepless nights, bonding with our baby, and trying to figure this nursing thing out. Even though it was hard, I was cherishing the moments of love that no one had ever been able to adequately describe to me.

At my follow-up appointment with my obstetrician, I pointed out the spot on my breast again. He casually recommended I just "keep an eye on it" again and check back in, if, in a couple weeks, nothing had changed. He assured me we could order an ultrasound if it were still there. Before I left, I noticed that my blood test results were normal except for one. I did not know what it was, but it was clearly out of range. Anxious and uncertain about what was happening, I insisted on a referral to figure it all out.

Within a few days, I was seen by a radiologist and what started out as an appointment for a breast ultrasound evolved into an order for a mammogram and then a biopsy. I received the results just a day after that.

The phone call came in the middle of my workday; I had an irregular, high-density mass in the left breast that was malignant. In layman's terms: it was breast cancer. As I put down the phone and tried to take in what I had just been told, I felt like I had been punched in the gut. Everything just stopped and for a moment, I almost forgot how to move. I mentally rewound all the times I had brought up the hard spot to healthcare professionals and been dismissed. I wanted to walk back into that office, months earlier and just shake them. As panic rose up in the back of my throat, all I could think was, *Why hadn't I advocated harder for myself?* My doctor called, saying he was so sorry for the diagnosis, and my immediate impulse was to hang up on him because he had been wrong. I wanted to scream into the phone, "I told you something was wrong, but you didn't listen!!!" I had trusted him.

I sat on the edge of my chair, contemplating how I could ever forgive him for the misdiagnosis as shock slowly took over. My son was only three months old; we were supposed to be going through all the three-month-old things right now; sleep regressions, smiles, tummy time. This period of life was supposed to be exhaustingly exciting as we soaked up our little guy. Instead, I was staring blankly at my computer screen, the weight of a cancer diagnosis sinking in.

* * *

On the first day back to work from maternity leave, while most new mothers might be catching up on emails or easing into their new working mom routine, I was now contemplating how to tell my boss I had cancer. I didn't know what came next, but I knew I couldn't carry it alone. I took a deep breath and dialed, and after a few rings, my new boss answered with a chipper, "Hey, welcome back! How's motherhood going?" We had known each other for years, but we had never worked together in this capacity. It took me a minute to gather the courage to respond; my voice trembled slightly, and I ignored all his questions and just blurted out, "I have breast cancer!" I tried to explain the situation, keep it simple, stick to just the facts, and eliminate the drama. But the moment the words left my mouth, silence followed for a long beat. And then his voice came, soft but steady, "I'm so, so sorry." The kindness in his tone caught me off guard—I didn't expect so much warmth. "You don't have to worry about anything here," he continued. "If working helps, we'd love to have you. If it doesn't, that's okay too. We'll make it work. We will carry you through this—until it's gone," he said, representing not only himself, but the organization's supportive position. I didn't realize I'd been holding my breath until I let it out. "And if you do work," he said, "don't force it on the hard days.

Turn it off when you need to. This work will still be here when you're ready." It wasn't a speech. It wasn't reassurance. It was a lifeline. In a season when my world felt like it was unraveling, he offered me space, grace, and the freedom to heal without fear of being forgotten.

For the first time in my life, I had no choice but to surrender to the help of others. In the past, I had never wanted to ask for help because I figured others needed more help than I did. I was capable and strong. I could do it, and help them too. But not this time. I was the one who needed the help and I knew I would not be able to survive this thing alone. I decided to work, and my colleagues fulfilled their promises by carrying me through. They sent meals, cards of encouragement, flowers, prayers, and offered me flexibility throughout the workday. I started to view every form of support as healing.

* * *

As expected, my first chemo treatment was highly nerve-wracking, although I walked into the infusion room with quiet confidence because I seemed younger than most in those chairs. Unknowingly, I had confused my age with the level of health. My nurse smiled as she hooked the line into my port, her movements practiced and gentle. I nervously smiled back, thinking confidently, *I can do this*, as I watched the fluid run down the line straight into the port on the upper-right side of my chest. About twenty minutes into it, my dad joined my husband and best friend in the infusion room with me. He had driven four hours to surprise me. He told me that he had tried to go to work that day, but his boss could tell he was extremely anxious and encouraged him to go and be with me. As a mother, I understood his anxiety. There is something about laying eyes on your child that strengthens us as parents, knowing they are okay; similarly, as children, seeing our parents in critical moments like these brings immediate calm. Even though the chemo running into my body was cold as ice, my heart was warm as I surveyed my support team, basking in the love and prayers of everyone thinking about me.

I can do this. I reassured myself again as I settled into the chemo chair. But a few hours later, I was on the bathroom floor, curled against cold tile, my forehead pressed against the floor, hoping it would provide some relief in between the waves of relentless nausea that wracked my body. A body that was in revolt—rejecting everything, including water. *I don't want to do this*, was all I could think. Groaning out loud, half-laughing in between dry heaves, I wondered how people survive getting drunk.

Time blurred for a moment until my body caught up with the anti-nausea medication, and I was okay . . . enough. It didn't take long for me to realize chemo wasn't just here to strip my strength; it was going to humble me too. I understood I had to survive cancer, but now, I realized I had to survive chemo too. In between bouts of mind altering sickness, I started to learn the rhythm. I kept a journal, not for soul-filled reflection, but to chart my survival. I carefully recorded the meds that worked and the foods that stayed down. I tracked which hours brought the worst of it on so I could prepare myself as best as possible. I learned when sleep was nonnegotiable and when I could steal everyday moments, like waking up in the middle of the night to feed our son. On those nights, I'd tiptoe into the nursery, shaky but determined to realize this experience with him. He never knew his mama had just come from battle. And because I had fought so hard, I never wanted to miss the quiet miracle of being there in the quiet of the night with him in my arms.

After four treatments, the faces in the infusion room began to feel familiar; the same women sat in the same recliners every Wednesday.

We quietly waged our own version of war within our bodies, minds, and spirits, not really saying anything to one another. Our companions, sisters, husbands, and friends sat next to us to support what was to come that day. At first, we exchanged glances. Then those looks became soft hellos and acknowledgements that said, "You're here again?" One woman, and her husband, always got the conversation going; we'd share our cancer stories and how we were handling the side effects of chemo. We'd crack jokes to lighten the mood; one woman said out loud what we were all thinking: "Hey, thank goodness we all have beautiful round heads because this baldness would not look good on us if we didn't!" After that, the energy in the room shifted on those Wednesdays. What was once a sterile and solemn environment became a friendly gathering for us all. We came from everywhere, and our stories were all different. One woman was dealing with her second round of breast cancer almost two decades apart. Four other women were dealing with their first round of breast cancer like me. Some of the women were still working, some were not, and then another woman, who was my age, was dealing with postpartum breast cancer too.

We even gave each other nicknames like we were a part of some unofficial club. Once, I misunderstood one of my fellow warriors' names for Karen, and so for the entire six months of treatment, I unknowingly called her Karen when her name was actually Vicky. That sweet woman allowed me to call her Karen the whole time because she understood what it felt like not to feel well and thought maybe I was losing my mind while on chemo. She did not have the heart to correct me. Boy, did we laugh when I realized my mistake. My nickname was "Lunchbox" because I brought an entire cooler bag of snacks to every treatment. I would bring enough to share, but many of the women did not find food appealing. It became a running joke. "What's on the Lunchbox menu today?" someone would ask before even sitting down.

As our friendship grew, our stories became more genuine. We continued to share tricks for managing nausea and other side effects. There was a comfort in the predictability of it all because our lives and the outcome of those lives were so unpredictable. In a place built for survival, we created a community of survivors. As the weeks passed and the treatment countdown grew smaller, we began to whisper our wonderings about life after and our plans for next steps. A collective hope bubbled beneath the fatigue and we signed a silent pact that we'd all make it to the finish line together. Who knew that the infusion room—a sterile box filled with beeping machines and fluorescent lights—could become a place of laughter, solidarity, and something startlingly close to joy. It was like God was trying to make the unbearable . . . bearable.

During those months of chemo, I started to reflect on what I could do to help my body stay strong as I was poisoning it with toxic chemicals. I had heard one of my Wednesday Chemo Sisters talk about the effectiveness of acupuncture and so I decided to give it a try. It had proved helpful in mitigating side effects like nausea and increasing energy. I would need help with both, so why not give it a try, I decided. I saw the same practitioner weekly, and we started to develop a friendship. They encouraged me to explore other approaches to maintain my body's strength, such as gratitude. As I considered the many people who supported us, I wanted them to know how grateful we were for their kindness. I started writing thank you cards to everyone who sent anything our way. Thank you card after thank you card created this excitement to express my gratitude within me, and I couldn't wait to send the next one. I shared this newfound joy I was experiencing in this practice with my acupuncturist during a session, and they were not surprised. "Yes, there are tremendous healing benefits available to us when we express gratitude," my acupuncturist confirmed. Who knew that writing thank you cards could have such a healing impact? I felt this was the start of something I could do to help my body stay strong, even if it was just from the emotional side. After exploring this notion of gratitude further, I started to incorporate the practice in different forms daily. I started small, like the thank you cards, and I journaled all the positive things that happened that day or that were in my life. Stepping into another day became exciting for me as I looked for things to be grateful for.

I'm grateful to be able to hug my husband and hold my son.
I'm grateful I can sit in the yard and breathe the fresh air.
I'm grateful for the family and friends all around me.

Noticing the simple things and letting the joy wash over me became a regular part of my day.

Little by little, my perspective on cancer began to change. I stopped seeing it as a challenge and started thinking of it as an opportunity. I was going to have hard days, sure, and I knew I would be faced with unplanned or unwanted news along the way, but because of this new outlook, I was able to reframe situations in my life in a way that was empowering. As I embraced social support and incorporated the practice of gratitude, I deeply embraced my relationships and loved more fiercely. I celebrated the final chemo by having my family and closest girlfriends in the chemo room join me, celebrating with me as I rang the bell, the symbol of triumph and closure over this treatment. This monumental moment was followed by a party to thank everyone who had carried us through it all. It was as beautiful as it was healing.

Life resumed as usual for the next couple of years, and I went back to living a mundane yet enjoyable existence. I went back to the things I liked to do, like raising a baby who was quickly entering the busy toddler stage and spending long pool days basking in the hot

Texas sun. I went on date nights with my husband and got together with friends and family for barbecues.

It was one of these gloriously regular afternoons, while lying down to get my eyebrows waxed, that I felt a sharp, stabbing pain in my back. A cold sense of dread washed over me as I assured myself that it was nothing. "I must be getting old!" I said out loud to the eyebrow lady with a laugh as I massaged the throbbing spot. But after weeks of using a foam roller, continuous stretching, and trying all sorts of topical creams to help try to alleviate the pain, I knew something else was going on. The pain didn't budge. I finally picked up the phone and scheduled the appointment.

As the doctor probed around on my back to see where I was sensitive to touch, she asked, "Where is the pain located? Out of zero to ten, how would you rate the pain? How often does the pain surface? Are you taking any over-the-counter medication to help with the pain?" It was after all of the questions that the oncologist decided, out of an "abundance of caution," to send me for a bone scan.

The results showed spots that they referred to as "suspicious." A CT scan was ordered, revealing another suspicious spot in the middle of my chest behind the ribs that then required an MRI, which led to further evaluation through a PET scan. It was at that follow-up appointment a few weeks later that my fears were all confirmed: The cancer was back, and it was metastatic.

On the drive home, my eyes were so blurred by my tears that I almost had to pull over. I gripped the steering wheel and put the car in auto-drive mode to ensure I stayed between the lines and in my lane. My mind went over everything I had done over the last few years that was supposed to prevent the recurrence of cancer. I had followed the posttreatment plan and then some, which was supposed to work, wasn't it? What did I miss? Did I not try hard enough? I knew I had done everything I could. I had followed the diet, incorporated exercise, managed my stress, and took the posttreatment drugs. Everyone I knew who had gone through cancer before me was okay, so why wasn't I?

After I recovered from the shock of the news and was able to silence all the noise around me, temporarily anyway, I gave myself time to accept the reality of the diagnosis and did my best to surrender it to God every morning. It was easy to trust God when things were going according to plan. Now, it was time to trust God with the biggest challenge of my life and that would take a commitment to daily practices. I started to piece together a plan, a roadmap to healing, over the next few months. Looking back, I can see now that cultivating this map gave me a sense of control in an otherwise uncontrollable situation. As the casualness of life continued to be stripped away I wanted to start living my life very intentionally from now on. I didn't know what I needed, but I knew this was a life and death decision and whatever practices I put in place would need to be empowering. My decision was confirmed when I was waiting at a doctor's office and a woman I didn't know stopped by me on her way out. She stopped so abruptly that I thought she had tripped, but as I looked closer, it seemed as if something was physically pulling her back, but no one was there. She looked me dead in the eye and said, "Sweetie, I don't know you, I don't know what you're going through, but the Holy Spirit sure did just tell me to stop and tell you that whatever it is: Focus, Fight, and Finish! And, you'll be all alright, so know that and do that!" And then she walked on. It was at that moment that I was empowered to start my intention.

I've always been an organized person, whether it is at work or managing my family, so it is no surprise that my first step was outlining my strongest reasons for living. I wrote those down and put them where I could see them every day to keep them as my North Star.

My son.

My husband.

My family and friends.

Once again, I welcomed the calls, cards, notes, texts of encouragement, and any help anyone offered. Every notion of help from parents, family, friends, and beyond felt like little drops of energy filling me up. I had long since established a workout routine, but I decided to visit with an integrative physical therapist to see where I could make tweaks and improve my overall physical fitness as I continued to fight cancer. I knew there was something I could do to refine my routine.

I revisited my diet and nutrition by referencing the work I had started with a dietitian just over a year before to ensure it aligned with the recommended nutrients and cancer-fighting foods. What I thought would be a quick review of my diet turned into an opportunity to lay the foundation for approaching the rest of the plan. I went through the dietitian program a few times, as she emphasized a phase-in approach to change. One meal at a time, then one day at a time, and then one week at a time, I added to my arsenal of weapons with broccoli and kale. This approach allowed transformation in my diet without me even really noticing it. It became a lifestyle over time, and because of that, it was surmountable. While it was my nutritionist that initially encouraged me to stop and turn around, so I could see how far I had come, I applied it to all the other areas of my life that I was approaching with more gentle attention and intention. One by one, the bricks were laid that formed the path to my healing. Slowly, I carved out time to meet my physical, spiritual, and emotional needs for whatever they needed in that day.

I continued my practice of gratitude, and because I had done it over the years, it was easy for me to strengthen it after I accepted where I was in life and turned it over to God. I almost immediately started making time for daily positive visualizations, picturing myself cured and healthy, repeating positive affirmations, in addition to having devotional time, as I began my day. "Every day, I am getting better," I would declare as I crawled out of bed and slowly walked to the shower. After some time I grew bolder in my journal writing and declared to heaven and earth, "I am healed, I am whole, and I am cured." The positive affirmations came to mind often throughout the day too. Whether I was driving down a road or looking in the rearview mirror at a stop light, repeating this phrase as many times as possible allowed me to shift my mindset from accepting that I had metastatic cancer to empowering myself by knowing what was in my body so I could pivot my actions when needed. This shift in perspective powerfully changed my energy and how I lived life in the moment. Not only did I love more fiercely, but I also started to live life more boldly and no longer shied away from doing things I wanted to do or saying things that needed to be said. If I had an opinion, good or bad, about a person, place, or thing, I shared it lovingly. I spoke up more when, in the past, I would have waited to be called on. If I had a desire to do something, I did it. I started responding to the nudges of people being laid on my heart and reaching out to them. I began appreciating experiences versus things. It was liberating. I saw myself as healed, believed myself as healed, and lived my life as healed.

* * *

I am optimistic by nature, but this newfound way of living created even more positivity in my life. I started to find new activities that brought joy to my household; I got certified in laughter yoga and trained as a floral designer, sharing my colorful creations with others. To maintain this positivity and joy, I also realized that what I watched, read, listened to, and consumed could dramatically influence my outlook on my healing journey and just my life overall. I evaluated everything in my life and worked to remove those things that created negativity so I would not be brought down. It was a life-or-death situation, and I knew it. What was once such a limiting experience with only two paths morphed into a garden of opportunity to try new things, if I just stayed open. I connected with an integrative care center to once again see what else I could be doing to keep my body as healthy and strong as possible to allow the oral chemo to do its job. They provided a complimentary herbal supplement protocol that would enhance treatment, help combat disease, and keep the body as strong as possible. I also learned the importance of incorporating stress management techniques, which created more confidence in managing the day-to-day of what I encountered and filled my healing bucket.

The last piece of my healing roadmap was the toughest. I knew there was emotional healing that needed to take place, and for me, that included forgiveness. I figured the two years I had spent talking out my problems with my therapist would cover everything, yet, the diagnosis of metastatic cancer made me realize that I still had lingering resentment in my heart. I work in healthcare and know young women get breast cancer at a young age. *Why hadn't I spoken up more? Why didn't they do more?* I realized I was grieving the loss of feeling safe, which had been taken from me at a time when I most needed it. *How was I going to come back from this?* I knew I needed to work through my anger again, so I talked to someone to help me identify the feelings that were lingering. There was hard emotional work ahead, but I was willing to face all the what-ifs because I had a sense of urgency to get all the anger and resentment out of my body. I wanted to live.

Taking time to think, I wrote honest letters to my care team for not acting sooner, and allowed myself grace for not speaking up, which was hugely healing. The forgiveness work that I thought I had done in other areas of my life had to be revisited all over again, and this time, it was deeper. This complex and painful work restored my life.

After a year of treatment, I was feeling great. But eventually, there was a progression, so I had to change treatment. There was anxiety in that, but it served as an opportunity to revisit the plan, review what I had been able to incorporate and refine it based on new information. I had learned to accept that my life would have ups and downs, so my goal was to move onward and upward despite those dips that would come my way.

Given my newfound lease on life, my husband and I embraced the mindset that if I expected to be healed, I would live a life as if I were healed. This mentality meant praying for an opportunity to continue growing our family. We decided it was time to walk down the path we had started years before after I was first in remission—surrogacy. I spoke with several women who continued to expand their family beyond their diagnosis, even when their cancer had metastasized. We understood the pros and cons of our situation, so we decided that the most significant thing was transparency and openness with a future surrogate. Almost two months after we decided to continue down the surrogacy path, we were matched with a family, and they were perfect. We quickly embraced each other's families, and they accepted the fact that I was living with cancer. The process moved by like a river current, swift, steady, and sacred, and then, just one year later, I held our second son for the first time. I felt as if our hearts were connected with his weight in my arms and his breath against my chest. My first son saved me and anchored me during the storm. This little one? He cracked open a new life.

As my story continues, I will always live with a metastatic disease. This healing plan has become more than my survival map; it has become my love story, built out of steady devotion to my life. With any grand plan or love story, things can sometimes go off course and require attention as it drifts, demanding recentering. So I return to it often, like before every scan, or during quiet moments of prayer, when something inside me whispers, *Look again*. I review, refine, and realign. Not just to stay alive but to stay deeply intentional here. Intentional living and my healing plan have transformed the way I inhabit my body, my mind, and my spirit. I once felt scattered, like my inner parts were speaking different languages, unable to communicate with each other, pulling me in opposing directions. The way I live now is filled with quiet, steady alignment. There is harmony and ease in my days, which I didn't know was possible, but has become the song of my life, even when the beat of a survivor's drum is clanging in the background. None of this means I'm untouched by life's chaos, but I'm no longer undone by it.

My radical expression of love is the unglamorous, daily work of staying alive and choosing to be here fully as a wife, a mother, a daughter, a sister, a cousin, and a friend. It's in God's love that I trust, and because of that, I have been able to navigate this precarious life for these last five years. There was a time when I didn't know how to do that. But when I came face-to-face with death, something innate and tender within me awakened. Love, I learned, isn't a thing you earn or prove. It's what you return to when everything else is stripped away. It's your oxygen when you can't breathe, it's the fuel you need to build something beautiful out of the ashes. I realized that I spent so much of my time, before my diagnosis, walking through life empty-handed, but now, I have practices that ground me when the waves of panic and fear rise threatening to take me under. Gratitude isn't just a word; it's the way I reintroduce myself to the world each morning, it's my declaration that I am here, I am alive, and I am giving back all that I have been given. Forgiveness is no longer a lofty idea; it's the practice that softens a healed heart and gives me back to myself. Because of these tools, I don't feel like I'm drowning anymore; instead, I'm face up, feeling the sun, floating on the calm waves of life, supported by something greater than me.

Life is now the sound of both sons' laughter in the morning while starting the day, the family sandwich hugs, two boys in the middle, and my husband and I on the outside. Life is the sweet kisses of my husband in the morning on the days he leaves earlier than me. It's tears that come on spontaneously, springing not from sadness but from the fullness of feeling everything because I now know everything can be lost. It's to choose life fiercely, even when it's ordinary. To love so hard that staying becomes a revolutionary act. This is what living fully looks like. This is what healing feels like.

AUTHOR BIO

Andrea Ralls is living life with newfound boldness and gratitude after a metastatic diagnosis, embracing each moment with a renewed sense of purpose. Her evolution after breast cancer has deepened her faith, strengthened her resilience, and given her a profound appreciation for life's beauty. She believes in the power of love, healing, and transformation, seeing challenges as opportunities to grow and inspire others along the way.

She believes that God led a path for her that combined the healing powers of the natural world with the healing powers of advanced medicine. Knowing that God is the author of her story, Andrea continues to honor every gift He provides, especially her two sons, who are miracles in and of themselves. Through it all, Andrea has witnessed the presence of God in adversity, recognizing His strength, peace, and grace guiding her forward.

With a background in the healthcare space, Andrea understands the balance between science and self-care, integrating both into her daily life. She finds immense joy in time with her husband and two boys and cherishes the unwavering support and love of family and friends. Based in Austin, Texas, she continues to prioritize wellness, healing, meaningful connections, and the pursuit of a life fully and fiercely lived.

Connect with Andrea and follow her here:

Instagram: @RootedandRadiant_RallsRhythm;

YouTube: @RootedandRadiant_RallsRhythm;

Email: RootedandRadiant.RallsRhythm@gmail.com.

www.ingramcontent.com/pod-product-compliance
Lightning Source LLC
Chambersburg PA
CBHW022046020426
42335CB00012B/566